T0226894

Sport Psychiatry

Editors

SILVANA RIGGIO
ANDY JAGODA

PSYCHIATRIC CLINICS
OF NORTH AMERICA

www.psych.theclinics.com

Consulting Editor
HARSH K. TRIVEDI

September 2021 • Volume 44 • Number 3

ELSEVIER

1600 John F. Kennedy Boulevard ● Suite 1800 ● Philadelphia, Pennsylvania, 19103-2899

http://www.theclinics.com

PSYCHIATRIC CLINICS OF NORTH AMERICA Volume 44, Number 3
September 2021 ISSN 0193-953X, ISBN-13: 978-0-323-83592-3

Editor: Lauren Boyle
Developmental Editor: Diana Ang

Psychiatric Clinics of North America (ISSN 0193-953X) is published quarterly by Elsevier Inc., 360 Park Avenue South, New York, NY 10010-1710. Months of issue are March, June, September, and December. Business and Editorial Offices: 1600 John F. Kennedy Blvd., Suite 1800, Philadelphia, PA 19103-2899. Periodicals postage paid at New York, NY and additional mailing offices. Subscription prices are $338.00 per year (US individuals), $966.00 per year (US institutions), $100.00 per year (US students/residents), $406.00 per year (Canadian individuals), $499.00 per year (international individuals), $1024.00 per year (Canadian & international institutions), and $220.00 per year (international students/residents), $100.00 per year (Canadian & students/residents). Foreign air speed delivery is included in all *Clinics*' subscription prices. All prices are subject to change without notice. **POSTMASTER:** Send address changes to *Psychiatric Clinics of North America*, Elsevier Health Sciences Division, Subscription Customer Service, 3251 Riverport Lane, Maryland Heights, MO 63043. **Customer Service: 1-800-654-2452 (US). From outside the United States, call 1-314-447-8871. Fax: 1-314-447-8029. E-mail: journalscustomerservice-usa@elsevier.com (for print support)** and **journalsonlinesupport-usa@elsevier.com (for online support)**.

Reprints. For copies of 100 or more, of articles in this publication, please contact the Commercial Reprints Department, Elsevier Inc., 360 Park Avenue South, New York, New York 10010-1710. Tel.: 212-633-3874, Fax: 212-633-3820, E-mail: reprints@elsevier.com.

Psychiatric Clinics of North America is covered in *MEDLINE/PubMed (Index Medicus), Current Contents/Social and Behavioral Sciences, Social Science Citation Index, Embase/Excerpta Medica,* and PsycINFO.

Contributors

CONSULTING EDITOR

HARSH K. TRIVEDI, MD, MBA
President and Chief Executive Officer, Sheppard Pratt Health System, Baltimore, Maryland, USA

EDITORS

SILVANA RIGGIO, MD
Professor, Department of Psychiatry, Neurology, Rehabilitation and Performance Medicine, Icahn School of Medicine at Mount Sinai, New York, New York, USA

ANDY JAGODA, MD
Professor and Chair Emeritus of Emergency Medicine, Emergency Medicine, Icahn School of Medicine at Mount Sinai, New York, New York, USA

AUTHORS

SHAILESH ADVANI, MD, PhD
National Institutes of Health, Bethesda, Maryland, USA

PIERRE BEAUCHAMP, PhD
Pro Hockey Analytics

DAVID CONANT-NORVILLE, MD
Mind Matters, PC, Hillsboro, Oregon, USA

SHANE A. CREADO, MD
Chicago, Illinois, USA

ALAN CURRIE, MB ChB, MPhil, FRCPsych
Consultant Psychiatrist, Cumbria Northumberland Tyne and Wear NHS Foundation Trust, Regional Affective Disorders Service, Wolfson Research Centre, Campus for Ageing and Vitality, Newcastle, United Kingdom; Mental Health Expert Panel (MHEP), English Institute of Sport, The Manchester Institute of Health and Performance, Manchester, United Kingdom; Visiting Professor, Department of Sport and Exercise Science, University of Sunderland, City Campus, Sunderland, United Kingdom

CARLA D. EDWARDS, MSc, MD, FRCP(C)
Assistant Clinical Professor, Department of Psychiatry and Behavioural Neuroscience, McMaster University, Hamilton, Ontario, Canada; High Performance Mental Health High Performance Mental Health Advisor: Swimming Canada, Cycling Canada, President: International Society for Sports Psychiatry

R. SHEA FONTANA, DO
Assistant Professor, Department of Psychiatry and Behavioral Health, University of South Carolina School of Medicine - Greenville, Prisma Health – Upstate, Greenville, Carolina, USA

IRA GLICK, MD
Professor Emeritus, Department of Psychiatry and Behavioral Sciences, Stanford University School of Medicine, Stanford, California, USA

PAUL H. GROENEWAL, PsyD
Inspire Wellness, Glen Rock, New Jersey, USA

AARON S. JECKELL, MD
Voluntary Faculty, Department of Psychiatry and Behavioral Health, Vanderbilt University School of Medicine, Nashville, Tennessee, USA

DANIELLE KAMIS, MD
Clinical Instructor, Department of Psychiatry and Behavioral Sciences, Stanford University School of Medicine, Voluntary Staff, Stanford University, Stanford, California, USA

LISA MACLEAN, MD
Henry Ford Health System, Detroit, Michigan, USA

DAVID R. McDUFF, MD
Clinical Professor of Psychiatry, University of Maryland School of Medicine, Baltimore, Maryland, USA; Maryland Centers for Psychiatry, Ellicott City, Maryland, USA

ERIC MORSE, MD
Carolina Performance, Raleigh, North Carolina, USA

ADENA NEGLIA, MS, RDN, CDN
Senior Dietitian, Brown & Medina Nutrition, New York, New York, USA; Director of Nutrition, Performance 360, Mount Sinai, New York, USA

MARISSA R. NORMAN, PsyD
Inspire Wellness Glen Rock, New Jersey, USA

DANIEL P. PERL, MD
Professor of Pathology (Neuropathology), Department of Pathology, F. Edward Hébert School of Medicine, Uniformed Services University of the Health Sciences, Bethesda, Maryland, USA

ROSEMARIE PERRY, PhD
Social Creatures, Department of Applied Psychology, New York University, Brooklyn, New York, USA

DEEPAK PRABHAKAR, MD, MPH
Sheppard Pratt, Baltimore, Maryland, USA

DAVID S. PRIEMER, MD
Assistant Professor of Pathology, F. Edward Hébert School of Medicine, Uniformed Services University of the Health Sciences, Henry M. Jackson Foundation for the Advancement of Military Medicine, Bethesda, Maryland, USA

ROSEMARY PURCELL, BA, MPsych, PhD
Head, Elite Sport and Mental Health, Orygen, Professorial Fellow and Deputy Head of Department, Centre for Youth Mental Health, The University of Melbourne, Parkville, Victoria, Australia

DAVID PUTRINO, PT, PhD
Assistant Professor, Department of Rehabilitation and Human Performance, Icahn School of Medicine at Mount Sinai, New York, New York, USA

SILVANA RIGGIO, MD
Professor, Department of Psychiatry, Neurology, Rehabilitation and Performance Medicine, Icahn School of Medicine at Mount Sinai, New York, New York, USA

SHARON BAUGHMAN SHIVELY, MD, PhD
Independent Researcher, Potomac, Maryland, USA

MEGAN E. SOLBERG, MA
Doctoral Candidate, Department of Counseling Psychology, Morgridge College of Education, University of Denver, Denver, Colorado, USA

MURRAY B. STEIN, MD, MPH
Distinguished Professor of Psychiatry and Public Health, University of California San Diego, Veterans Affairs San Diego Healthcare System, La Jolla, California, USA

TODD STULL, MD, DFAPA
Clinical Associate Professor, Department of Psychiatry and Neuroscience, University of California, Riverside, School of Medicine, Riverside, California, USA

VUONG VU, MD
Mind Matters, PC, Hillsboro, Oregon, USA

Contents

The field of Sport Psychiatry is in early stages of development and the role of the sport psychiatrist continues to evolve as the psychiatric needs of athletes become more apparent. Today's sports psychiatrist has increasing roles, including treatment of athletes, coaches, and their support personnel as well as providing an in depth and broad understanding of the medical and psychiatric demands in sport. The ongoing development of the field will help determine the eventual growth and expansion in the field.

Many factors place athletes at increased risk of compromised performance, including mental health symptoms and disorders. Mental health disorders are common among athletes and if untreated may impair outcomes. Cultural influences including social media, negative attitudes about help seeking mental help, and stereotyping, when not addressed, compromise a healthy wholesome training environment that may limit outcomes. In addition to addressing mental health needs, cultural influencers and barriers, specifically designed and targeted psychological skills to assist with performance are reviewed. These skills can promote mental toughness and resiliency and can to higher levels of confidence and achievement.

This review presents a conceptual framework of burnout using models that have been developed throughout the years and provides the basis for the psychological measures used in clinical evaluations. Clinical gold standards, including the Athlete Burnout Questionnaire and the Maslach Burnout Inventory, are reviewed, compared, and contrasted. Because many of the interventional approaches to burnout are centered around the concept of motivation, organizational interventions are proposed using Self-Determination Theory and other models that promote motivation.

Athletes may first seek counsel from mental health professionals with concerns of performance anxiety. The mental health professional must carefully explore the context and origins of the athlete's anxiety in order to identify and address the root cause. A detailed history and physical examination will help avoid missing comorbid conditions presenting with anxiety symptoms. This chapter highlights the importance of recognizing the circumstances in which anxiety symptoms may arise in athletes; identifying stressors that are exclusive to the athlete experience; determining how those symptoms can affect their performance and general livelihood; and developing a treatment strategy that maximizes the athlete's performance.

Major depressive disorder and other related disturbances in mood account for the highest proportion of psychiatric illnesses in the general population and are a leading cause of disability around the world. Despite belief to the contrary, athletes are vulnerable to the same mental illnesses as the general population. Unique circumstances experienced by athletes create challenges that are exclusive to that population, which can place them at greater risk for depression and other mental illnesses. This chapter explores the incidence of depression and related mood disturbances in athletes, risk factors for illness, obstacles to assessment and management, and treatment strategies.

Healthy sleep behaviors are a cornerstone to mental wellness and sports performance among athletes. Disturbances in sleep timing, quantity, and quality may impact an athlete's performance in the short and long term. Sleep disturbances may contribute to overall health, risk of injury, and career duration. This review discusses the prevalence of sleep disorders among athletes and its impact on mental health problems. A strategic approach is provided and highlights the importance of proactively identifying sleep disorders versus waiting for the problem to express itself. A summary of available therapeutic interventions to improve sleep in the athlete population is presented.

The pressure to gain mass, power, explosiveness, and endurance and to obtain a performance edge continues to a part of sports. Anabolic agents, including selective androgen receptor modulators along with peptides, hormones, and metabolic modulators, continues to evolve. Methods to promote transcription to modify gene expression are a part of the evolution. In order to monitor and improve doping detection, the Athlete Biological Passport has been created. This article provides an up-to-date review of alcohol, anabolic androgens and related agents, stimulants, opioids, and cannabis and related compounds and their effects on athlete health and performance.

Attention-deficit/hyperactivity disorder (ADHD), characterized by inattention, impulsivity and hyperactivity is a major health problem. This paper discusses ADHD across the life span and looks at the impact of debilitating symptoms, diagnosis, and treatment in athletes. Psychosocial interventions, with or without psychopharmacology including stimulants and non-stimulants, are discussed to help athletes achieve their highest level of symptom abatement and functioning. The age of the patient, the sport played, the athlete's overall health, and the regulations of the sport-governing body play a role in determining the most appropriate treatment.

This article provides an overview of the nutrition requirements for athletes, and gives insight into why this is often an area of confusion for both the athletic community and the general population. In addition, the prevalence of eating disorders and disordered eating in athletes is reviewed, and how and why they may go unnoticed. In addition, a discussion is provided on the harmful effects of unhealthy food behaviors on health and performance, and how to assess and establish a care team for an athlete who is struggling.

This article focuses on neuropsychiatric clinical expression and neuropathology associated with chronic traumatic encephalopathy (CTE), which is thought to develop years after traumatic brain injury. The incidence, prevalence, additional risk factors, and pathophysiology remain largely unknown. CTE is considered a tauopathy because the endogenous brain protein tau, in its hyperphosphorylated state (p-tau), defines the predominant neuropathological findings and may underlie aspects of cell toxicity, synapse and circuit dysfunction, and clinical signs and symptoms. We discuss pathophysiological mechanisms possibly affecting p-tau accumulation. Finally, we interweave how clinical features and neuroanatomical sites associated with CTE potentially intersect with posttraumatic stress disorder.

Neurobehavioral sequelae after mild traumatic brain injury are multifactorial, often necessitating a multidisciplinary approach. Neurobehavioral sequelae generally resolve within 3 months; when more persistent, a search for contributing factors beyond a brain injury should be done. To accomplish this, a systematic and comprehensive evaluation is recommended to place the complaint in context of the patient's premorbid state. The treatment of neurobehavioral sequelae cannot be accomplished without a clear understanding of the underlying cause, and the treatment must be placed within a patient's social and functional framework. Normalizing the experience through education of patients and their families facilitates recovery.

Aaron S. Jeckell and R. Shea Fontana

Participation in youth sport is not without the potential for risk including exposure to injury and sport-related concussion (SRC). SRC is an injury that disproportionately affects active youths and carries with it numerous psychological, social, and biological implications. This article aims to (1) examine the scope of the problem that SRC poses for the athletic community, (2) explore the social impact that SRC and media portrayal of this injury has, (3) discuss how this may affect an athlete who has experience SRC and efforts to return to activity, (4) and evaluate a meaningful way to navigate all of these factors with athletes who experience SRC.

David Putrino, Paul H. Groenewal, and Rosemarie Perry

One important element for forming and cultivating a high performing team in any sport is player selection. For most professional sports, this is an intense period whereby coaching, performance, and administrative staff must work together and use collective wisdom to identify players who have the best probability of consistent high performance. The stakes of a draft are high: the wrong choice can be incredibly costly and impact a team's performance and culture for many years. This article identifies and details common features of the drafting procedure, followed by a discussion of best practices for structuring and executing a draft protocol.

Alan Currie and Rosemary Purcell

Athletes commonly experience mental health symptoms. However, prevalence estimates require refinement so that symptoms are interpreted in context and diagnostic labels are accurately applied. Further prevalence studies are also needed in subgroups within sport, in particular female athletes, athletes with disabilities, and coaches. Existing consensus-based and evidence-based therapies must be adapted not only to the individual athlete but also to the ecology of sports. Filling the gaps in our knowledge on what treatment modifications may be required for the individual athlete and how services should be designed to deliver treatment most effectively will require well-designed studies that use standardized terminology and defined outcome measures.

PSYCHIATRIC CLINICS OF NORTH AMERICA

SERIES OF RELATED INTEREST

Child and Adolescent Psychiatric Clinics of North America
https://www.childpsych.theclinics.com/

Neurologic Clinics
https://www.neurologic.theclinics.com/

THE CLINICS ARE AVAILABLE ONLINE!
Access your subscription at:
www.theclinics.com

Preface

The Mind-Body Interface: Maximizing Peak Performance

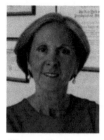 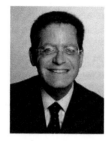

Silvana Riggio, MD   Andy Jagoda, MD
Editors

It is with great pleasure that we accepted the role of coeditors for this issue of the *Psychiatric Clinics of North America* on Sport Psychiatry. One of us (Silvana Riggio) is a Psychiatrist and a Neurologist and the other (Andy Jagoda) is an Emergency Medicine Physician. We have collaborated both clinically and academically over the past 35 years, sharing a strong interest in all aspects of sports medicine. We have worked with professional sports teams and with the military across the spectrum of care. Much of our work over the years has focused on traumatic brain injury, which provides an excellent model to demonstrate the importance of a multidisciplinary approach in caring for athletes; an approach that underscores the importance of education, prevention, acute care, and long-term sequelae management. Historically, athletes have received varying degrees of multidisciplinary care, although clinical experience from our different perspectives on health care systems suggests that the mental health side of care has not always been fully appreciated.

The mind-body interface impacts all facets of performance and recovery. Of paramount importance in the care of the athlete is both an understanding of the relationship between physical symptoms and psychological response and an understanding of the complex world the athlete lives in. It is only in recent years that this interface has been formally recognized in the sports world, and that mechanisms for integrating physical and mental health have been implemented. Sport Psychiatry is the discipline dedicated to maximizing performance through increasing awareness of one's physical and mental strengths and weaknesses and channeling the mind's contribution to physical performance. There is no demarcation between the two, but without coordinated strategies, an athlete may risk failure in achieving their full potential. In recognition of the importance of mental health in athletes, the International Olympic Committee convened a group of experts in 2018 to put forth a consensus statement on the mental

Psychiatr Clin N Am 44 (2021) xiii–xv
https://doi.org/10.1016/j.psc.2021.06.001
0193-953X/21/© 2021 Published by Elsevier Inc.

health in elite athletes.[1] That same year, the International Society of Sport Psychiatry published their first text on the field.[2]

The Sport Psychiatrist is well positioned to help the athlete and their health care team, not only when there is an acute problem but also as part of the health maintenance program that facilitates peak performance. The healthy athlete who has an in-depth understanding of why they do what they do can more easily find ways to augment the mental stamina needed to perform. Conversely, the injured athlete often deals with both physical and mental health challenges that must be recognized and addressed in order to expedite recovery. Physical rehabilitation strategies are key, but in order to be comprehensive, there must be a mental rehabilitation strategy… which is often overlooked, resulting in potentially negatives outcomes. An injury that can be considered minor for some may represent a source of great concern for an elite athlete, and without properly dealing with that concern, it may undermine recovery.

Mental performance and physical performance are on a two-way street, each dependent on the other. Comprehensive care of the elite athlete requires assessing and monitoring a wide range of factors that are interrelated; beyond medical comorbidities, factors include personality structure, motivation, coping mechanisms, support structure, underlying primary psychiatric disorders, medications, alcohol and illicit drug use, sleep disturbances, and nutrition. At times, the athlete's mental health needs are compromised either because resources are not made available to them or because of other barriers, such as the stigma some hold against psychiatric care, social and family pressures, poor self-identity, and or the need for a "quick fix" without understanding the dedicated work often needed to address underlying issues. The Sport Psychiatrist is positioned to assess the athlete and understand the cultural background, sources of stress, and the relationship between medical and psychiatric comorbidities. They are able to evaluate and balance both the pharmacologic and the psychotherapeutic needs of the athletes; by optimizing the mental health of the athlete, maximal performance can be achieved.

The ability to focus on a task (attention) is a critical component for an athlete to reach their full potential. Anything that interferes with the athlete's ability to focus (eg, stress, anxiety, depression, drugs) will impact performance; if not recognized and treated accordingly, the athlete risks failure both on the field and off the field. Consequently, an ongoing dialog across all members of the health care team is necessary.

Our goal for this issue of *Psychiatric Clinics of North America* is to provide an up-to-date resource on Sport Psychiatry; to do so, we assembled a group of experts, many of whom are established international leaders in the field. Our hope is that this issue will facilitate communication between all members of the athlete's care team and emphasize the Sport Psychiatrist's role on that team. The science of Sport Psychiatry is still in its infancy; there are basic principles from the world of psychiatry that can be imported into the management of the athlete, but athletes, especially world-class competitors, are unique both physiologically and mentally. Their psychological and physical needs must be addressed early and monitored throughout their careers in order to help them reach and maintain their individual and/or teams' goals.

Silvana Riggio, MD
Icahn School of Medicine at Mount Sinai
One Gustave Levy Place
New York, NY 10029, USA

Andy Jagoda, MD
Icahn School of Medicine at Mount Sinai
One Gustave Levy Place
New York, NY 10029, USA

E-mail addresses:
silvana.riggio@mountsinai.org (S. Riggio)
andy.jagoda@mountsinai.org (A. Jagoda)

REFERENCES

1. Reardon C, Hainline B, Aron C, et al. Mental health in elite athletes: International Olympic Committee consensus statement (2019). Br J Sports Med 2019;53: 667–99.
2. Glick I, Stull T, Kamis D, editors. The ISSP manual of sports psychiatry. Oxfordshire, UK: Routledge Publisher; 2018. p. 294.

The Role of a Sport Psychiatrist on the Sports Medicine Team, Circa 2021

Todd Stull, MD[a],*, Ira Glick, MD[b], Danielle Kamis, MD[b,1]

KEYWORDS

- Sport Psychiatry • Sport Psychiatrist • Pharmacotherapy • Psychotherapy
- Sports domain

KEY POINTS

- Sport Psychiatry is a relatively new field that is evolving to meet the increasing mental health and psychiatric needs of athletes.
- The knowledge, skills, and abilities along with the needs of athletes, coaches, and their teams help define the role of the Sport Psychiatrist working within an integrated medical sports team. A Sport Psychiatrist needs to have a working knowledge of the roles and responsibilities of each of the members of the integrated sports team that supports athletes, coaches, and teams.
- Tools used by the Sport Psychiatrist include psychotherapy, pharmacotherapy, mental skills training, and combined treatment.
- The Sport Psychiatrist must understand pharmacokinetics, pharmacodynamics, and the athletic requirements needed to perform in athletic settings.
- Types of interventions and treatments provided require an understanding of the demands of the sport, athlete needs, and strategies to improve mental health and performance in safe and ethical ways.

INTRODUCTION

The role of Sport Psychiatry continues to develop, evolve, and become increasingly important in the world of sports. This has been driven by the shift in focus of the mental well-being of athletes. After gathering data from student athletes and finding the number 1 concern expressed was related to mental health and wellness, the National

Authors have no financial or commercial conflict of interests.
[a] Department of Psychiatry and Neuroscience, University of California Riverside, School of Medicine, UCR Health- Citrus Tower, 3390 University Avenue Suite 115, Riverside, CA, 92501, USA; [b] Department of Psychiatry and Behavioral Sciences, Stanford University School of Medicine, 401 Quarry Road, Stanford, CA, 94305, USA
[1] Present address: 164 Main Street Sui 201, Los Altos, CA 94022.
* Corresponding author.
E-mail address: Todd.stull@medsch.ucr.edu

Psychiatr Clin N Am 44 (2021) 333–345
https://doi.org/10.1016/j.psc.2021.04.001
0193-953X/21/© 2021 Elsevier Inc. All rights reserved.

Collegiate Athletic Association (NCAA) formed a mental health task force in 2014. *Mind, Body and Sport: Understanding and Supporting Student-Athlete Mental Wellness*[1] and *Interassociation Consensus Document: Best Practices for Understanding and Supporting Student-Athlete Mental Wellness*[2] Sports Science Institute of the NCAA; 2016. In 2016, the *International Review of Psychiatry* published a special issue focused on the field with a broad range of topics including its history, how a Sport Psychiatrist works with teams, psychiatric medications, and psychotherapy interventions as well as related topics, including cheating, performance enhancing drugs, concussion, and the culture of sports.[3] This publication was followed by the International Olympic Committee in 2018 convening a group of experts to put forth guidelines on "Mental Health In Elite Athletes."[4] In 2018, the International Society of Sport Psychiatry published the first text on the field. This text covered both individual sports, like skiing, and team sports, like basketball.[5]

This article describes the range of knowledge, skills, and abilities necessary to be a Sport Psychiatrist. It covers the Sport Psychiatrist's broad range of roles with a focus on the tools used to help an athlete, team, clubs, and coaches. Although not exhaustive, it provides an overview of mental illness treatment of specific disorders and strategies to optimize performance using mental skills.

THE SPORT PSYCHIATRY FIELD

Sports include all forms of competitive physical activity or competition in which training improves physical ability and mental skills. Part of the role of sports is to provide enjoyment and often entertainment. Sport provides an environment for skill acquisition and development. Beyond physical skill development, other benefits of sports include teamwork, communication, working toward goals, development of loyalty, commitment, and working through conflict. Sports create a setting to learn routines, develop composure, focus under stress, and build confidence. But most important, participation in a sport is an important part of the identity for many men, women, and children in most cultures around the world, for example, basketball in the United States, football (soccer) in European countries, or badminton in Thailand.

The first publication on Sport Psychiatry was written in 1967 by Arnold R. Beisser,[6] a psychiatrist, and then 20 years later by the physician J.H. Massamino.[7] Psychiatrist Begel and Burton[8] helped launch the field in the early 1990s. The field of Sport Psychiatry continues to develop and over the past several years has gained recognition and gradual understanding of what it does. Athletes who suffered from mental health problems were limited in options for evaluation and treatment. They may have been ignored or provided short and ineffective interventions by individuals with limited training in psychiatric illness.

The aims of the field of Sport Psychiatry are to evaluate, treat, and manage psychiatric symptoms or disorders in athletes and to optimize the mental health of athletes. The International Society for Sport Psychiatry is an organization whose goals are to implement the science and practice of psychiatry to the athletic community and to provide psychiatric and substance use evaluation and treatment, education, and research. The organization is focused on helping athletes enjoy the benefits of sports while managing their mental health. Additional roles of Sport Psychiatry are to address barriers, such as stigma, harassment, and lack of mental health literacy, along with cultural influences, including social media and negative attitudes about mental illness.

As the growth of the field advanced and sports continue to play an important role in culture, athletes who developed a mental illness have been offered an opportunity to continue their career by obtaining psychiatric treatment[5] As the intersection of psychiatric treatment and sports advances, appropriate and individualized mental health care must be prioritized. The nuances of a Sports Psychiatrist and their work with athletes have been expanded with a greater emphasis on the influence of gender, sexual orientation, race, and culture on the athlete's mental health.

Over the years and with the initiation of Title IV, female athletic participation has expanded in sports. A Sports Psychiatrist considers known gender-specific mental health care trends when evaluating and treating a female athlete. For example, it has been found that certain disorders, such as generalized anxiety disorder as well as major depressive disorder, are more prevalent in female athletes compared with their male counterparts. Additionally, mental health care concerns can fluctuate from sport to sport. For example, female athletes participating in aesthetic sports, such as gymnastics and figure skating, experience increased frequency of general anxiety disorder.[9] Moreover, the most common sports in which female athletes develop eating disorders are found in what are considered leanness sports, such as long-distance running, gymnastics, figure skating, and cheerleading. The incidence of eating disorders is strongly gender-dependent, and women are significantly more likely than men to have had anorexia or bulimia in their lifetime. Some studies put female incidence of eating disorders as high as 60% for highly competitive female athletes.[10]

Additionally, there exists gender-specific disorders, such as the female athletic triad, which involves simultaneously an eating disorder, menstrual irregularity, and reduction of bone density. Due to the complex nature of the triad, the Sport Psychiatrist uses a multidisciplinary approach, including a primary care physician, nutritionist, physical trainer, and the coaching staff. Furthermore, it is important that the psychiatrist understands that female athletes can be subjected to an alarming rate of sexual abuse. It is well known that sexual harassment in female athletes is a serious issue that additionally requires screening and must be evaluated and approached with sensitivity.

Furthermore, the Sports Psychiatrist must have not only an awareness of gender-specific treatment but also an understanding of an athlete's sexual orientation and sexual identity. At times, some heterosexual student athletes are in denial that team members are part of the lesbian, gay, bisexual, transgender, and queer or questioning (LGBTQ+) community and LGBTQ+ athletes may experience the burden of increased negative reactions from team members. This burden of discrimination appears to be a contributing factor to the elevated incidence of depression, alcohol and drug abuse, and suicide attempts in LGBTQ+ athletes. Comprehensive mental health care management by a Sport Psychiatrist can help address discrimination and its consequences.

Regarding minority athletes, a Sport Psychiatrist understands the importance of insight and understanding into an athlete's backgrounds and upbringing is critical. Many minority athletes have been subjected to racial profiling, which may lead to additional pressures and stressors that affect their mental health.

It important to understand the difficulties and blockades of minority athlete who are thrust into a new competitive athletic environment, especially in collegiate or professional sports. The Sport Psychiatrist plays a role to understand the minority perspective and be mindful that a period of adjustment and individualized treatment is appropriate.

Many athletes who experience a substance use disorder or other psychiatric disorder are not able to continue participating competitively. More athletes are matriculating to college and play a sport with a mental illness than ever in the history of sports. Having a mental illness once was a career-ending diagnosis—and now this not always is the case. An athlete's state of mind has an important impact on performance and participation in sports effects emotion, cognitions, behavior, and overall health. Psychiatric care of athletes, to be effective, incorporates both bio-psychosocial and cultural factors, and places them into the athlete's context. Sport Psychiatry pushes to protect the health of athletes and not ruin them for amusement. As the growth of the field of Sport Psychiatry continues to expand, the role of a Sport Psychiatrists evolves and addresses individual, family, team, parents, coaches, and the influence or roles of others. Delivery of treatment is based on the psychiatric disorder and presenting problem using a combination of modalities ranging from medication to psychotherapy to mental skills training to use of psychophysiology. More teams, coaches, and athletes now are recognizing the importance of early identification and treatment to address mental health symptoms and disorders to continue to train and compete. Sport Psychiatrists increasingly are involved in the treatment of substance use disorders. Although athletes and sports teams and organizations have been slow to accept treatment of psychiatric disorders, the tide is changing.[5,11]

THE ROLE OF THE SPORT PSYCHIATRIST

A Sports Psychiatrist is a fully trained physician who has attained specialty postgraduate training and experience in psychiatric and substance evaluations; they are trained in the treatment of emotional, cognitive, and behavioral symptoms seen in athletes. Most psychiatrists are board certified in psychiatry. There is an additional certification process for Sports Psychiatrists that represents the highest standard in the field. Sport Psychiatry is not recognized as a subspeciality by the Accreditation Council for Graduate Medical Education. A certification track is offered for psychiatrist who want to obtain additional qualifications through the International Society for Sport Psychiatry (https://www.sportspsychiatry.org). A Sports Psychiatrist has a broad range and depth of training and can provide a biopsychosocial and cultural formulation to care and deliver a full range of treatment options. The medical training of a Sports Psychiatrist provides a unique conduit between sports medicine and mental health providers and other members of the integrated sports team (IST) (**Fig. 1**). A Sports Psychiatrist often operates with a consultation and team (community) model to actively provide or lead in the implementation of shared care and management of treatment goals with other clinicians. Skills are applied, adapted, and contextualized specifically for developmental stages and settings ranging from beginning to high performance environments in sport. The central role of the psychiatrist is to provide clinical psychiatric

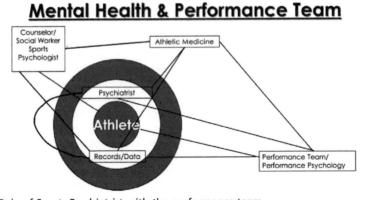

Fig. 1. Role of Sports Psychiatrist with the performance team.

care to the athletic community that is mutually dependent on athletic performance and health and well-being.

Importantly, the years of medical and psychiatric training that a Sports Psychiatrist has make their role very different from that of a nonphysician, such as psychologists, social workers, and nurses—who also have very specialized but different skills. The role of a Sport Psychiatrist is changing. **Fig. 2** represents the continuum of the range of roles of the psychiatrist in treating athletes from severe mental illness to athletes who are healthy but wish to learn specific skills to enhance performance.

Just as important as recognizing and describing the role, abilities needed, and the range of skills and knowledge in the field, likewise, it is increasingly important for a Sport Psychiatrist to understand and have a working knowledge of the roles of various individuals within the IST (**Fig. 3**). The IST (**Box 1**) is designed to work with individuals and teams within a given sport. Each sport has a unique set of requirements needed to excel and perform optimally. The psychiatrist is best equipped to have a working knowledge of the multidimensional nature of the athlete's life and the roles, responsibilities, terminology, and understanding of sports and how each individual or area functions. The Sport Psychiatrist needs to have a strategy to communicate within the IST and effectively implement it (see **Box 1**). Psychosomatic disorders, concussion, and psychiatric disorders that are substance induced or due to a medical disorder are examples where the skills and knowledge of a Sports Psychiatrist are unique. The Sport Psychiatrist plays a key role in the overtraining or paradoxic deconditioning syndrome. For example, overtraining can lead to underperformance, which may be misinterpreted that an athlete has depression. An athlete's lack of proper fueling can lead to inadequate energy and they may appear unmotivated or sluggish and thus the knowledge and skills to treat low energy availability conditions, such as the female triad/relative energy deficiency in sports are common for a Sports Psychiatrist. An athlete who is sleep deprived has impaired reaction time, diminished energy, impaired decision making under pressure, and impaired emotional control. These athlete data are tracked and monitored for each athlete on a weekly and monthly basis and compared with performance times as athletes approach World Cups and World Championships. Consequently, Sport Psychiatrists with data support can play a critical role in decision-making process regarding athlete health, well-being, and performance demands.

The Sport Psychiatrist can help a team/organization create a list of screening tools to use in identifying those athletes who may need further evaluation for a substance

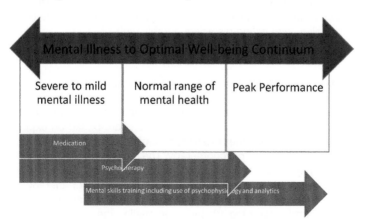

Fig. 2. Full continuum for Sport Psychiatrist working with athletes.

Internal Performance Model

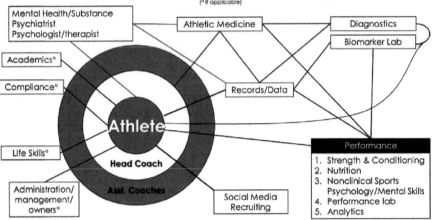

Fig. 3. Internal performance model of the IST for athletes.

use or psychiatric disorder. A part of this process ideally should include education to the stakeholders of an organization. Education helps create an understanding of mental health and substance-related issues and how they are identified, evaluated, treated, and managed. Education of athletes, teams, coaches, and so forth provides an opportunity to discuss prevention and rationale for prevention. The importance of preventative steps, such as proper sleep, nutrition, rest, and recovery, and the importance of trusting relationships and how to manage stress and access care, if needed, can make an impactful difference in the life of an athlete.[11]

The treatment approach always should start with a diagnostic evaluation and work-up to rule out medical causes for psychiatric symptoms and disorders. An integrated multidisciplinary treatment approach that includes psychotherapy coupled with psychopharmacotherapy if indicated should follow. The authors agree with the general guidelines of Currie and Johnston.[12]

The prevalence of mental health symptoms and disorders in elite athletes is approximately 34% for symptoms of anxiety and depression. Alcohol abuse is just under 20% in male athletes depending on the sport and culture, whereas in female elite athletes, depression and anxiety rates are thought to be higher than in male athletes, depending on several variables, with eating disorders notably high.

PSYCHOTHERAPY

Psychotherapy often is the treatment of choice for mental health symptoms and psychiatric disorders, depending on the severity. Pharmacotherapy is used and can be effective as well. Controlled scientific studies in athletes for both psychotherapy and pharmacotherapy are lacking, and recommendations are based on expert opinions, that is, clinical experience. Athletes often are disciplined and compliant and, therefore, can make good candidates for psychotherapy. The most common types of therapy for athletes include psychodynamic therapy, psychoeducation therapy, interpersonal psychotherapy, supportive psychotherapy, cognitive behavior therapy (CBT), and solution-focused therapy, with the occasional use of group or family therapy. The psychiatrist needs to understand the athlete's personality, the context of their situation, the sport, and the cultural influences. These factors assist in forming the therapeutic

---

Box 1
Athlete-centered roles of members of the integrated Sport Team for the Sport Psychiatrist

Strength and conditioning
  Metabolic circuits
  Movement patterns
  Training loads
  Periodization of training
  Rest and recovery strategies
  Monitoring and measuring

Nutrition
  Proper timing of fueling
  Weight management
  Body composition and changes
  Macronutrient, micronutrients, and trace elements
  Supplements
  Tracking body composition changes
  Body mapping/frame analysis for a sport or specific position

Analytics
  Monitor training (eg, sleep and performance within yearly training plan)
  Why they are used (eg, time series analysis of hormones, blood data, and performance)
  Data collected often relevant for the Sport Psychiatrist

Coaches
  Leadership and overall management of their team—roles and responsibilities for their team

Administration and management (eg, high performance director)
  Overall management and leadership for athletic program/organization

Athletic medicine
  Team physician/other physicians
  Athletic trainers
  Concussion management team

Academic staff and other support staff
  Assist with academic studies, tutors, and learning

Families, friends, and significant others
  Important roles in support and well-being in life of athlete

Psychologists or mental health professionals
  Provide psychotherapy and testing when indicated

Mental skills trainers
  Work with athletes and teams to implement psychological skills training to help with performance

Sports scientists (eg, physiologists and biomechanics)
  Focus on methods to assist with training, recovery from injury, and maximize physical capacity

---

relationship. It is the therapeutic relationship that is the key element for all types of psychotherapy with athletes. In addition, evidence-based treatment principles should be followed.

In the training and competition environment, athletes are used to having their progress measured, recorded, and evaluated. There has been a recent movement in athletics to measure the effects of psychotherapy. An outcome rating scale (ORS) evaluates personal well-being, interpersonal relationships, and social brief measure designed to assess the degree of severity of clients' experience in key areas of life functioning. The ORS specifically uses 4 four scales that measure individual personal well-being, interpersonal connections, social well-being, and overall well-being.

Individual psychotherapy can be helpful and used as an adjunct to medication. Psychoeducation is an imperative part of treatment. For mild depressive and anxiety systems and some adjustment issues, psychotherapy alone is often the treatment of choice. In the past, psychodynamic treatment and supportive psychotherapy have been the most common psychotherapy used. CBT has the most empirical support for the treatment of a variety of psychiatric conditions[13] and focuses on teaching athletes to recognize their thoughts, feelings, and behaviors and their associations.[14] CBT is a brief intervention treatment focused on teaching skills to manage, including situation-specific performance issues. CBT often resonates with athletes because it provides structure, goals, and direction via the manualized nature of the treatment. Dialectical behavioral therapy is a type of CBT that can be helpful for athletes who are experiencing interpersonal difficulties, emotional dysregulation, and inability to manage stress and who may benefit from mindfulness training.

Acceptance and commitment therapy (ACT) is another type of cognitive behavioral therapy and can be applied in sports to enhance performance and overall well-being of athletes. ACT is a mindfulness-based psychotherapy technique that focuses on an athlete's thoughts, feelings, and behavior and how they interact to influence their physiology and psychological well-being. ACT can be very helpful in the performance and overall energy management of athletes. Foundational ingredients to ACT include cognitive diffusion nonjudgmental acceptance, engaging the present moment, self-observation, and committed value-driven action.

Solution-focused therapy is focused on solving everyday life problems by finding solutions and empowering the athlete. Solution-focused therapy is based on the athlete being the expert, focusing on what works and the present with the idea there are exceptions, problems often only need small adjustments, and cooperation to achieve a solution.

Motivational enhancement therapy (MET) often is used for substance abuse and substance use disorders to assist the athletes with their ambivalent feelings toward substance use. It is based on the principles of motivation interviewing. MET has been shown to facilitate greater participation in treatment and remaining in treatment.

PHARMACOTHERAPY

Prescribing medication is based on the psychiatric diagnosis, prognostic evaluation, and severity of symptoms. The therapeutic alliance—focused the treatment relationship—is important to medication adherence. Clinical skills—like knowing how to combine medication with some form of psychotherapy—along with the psychiatrist-athlete relationship are import for monitoring and managing athletes who are treated with medication. It is important to stabilize an athlete's psychiatric disorder initially and manage any side effects while considering safety and return to training or competition. The psychiatrist should take into consideration the specific sport and position as well as its demands, biomedical conditions including pharmacokinetic and pharmacodynamic issues, and other health problems and medications the athlete may be taking. Other factors to be considered when prescribing medications to athletes include the therapeutic effects, positive or negative effects on performance, nontherapeutic performance enhancing effects, safety, and side effects. Medications are used more frequently in those athletes with more severe psychiatric illness like major depressive disorder, bipolar disorder, and/or schizophrenia but should be prescribed whenever indicated.

When treating psychiatric disorders in athletes, it must be understood that many disorders have genetic etiologies, cause severe dysfunction, and have to be treated over a lifetime. As such, even for athletes, the disorder must be treated to achieve efficacy to restore function. The side effects can be managed over time, when the athlete returns to competition.

There is limited evidence regarding medication treatment, and guidance comes primarily from extrapolation from general population recommendations, and from expert opinion regarding athlete prescribing. The most important issue is to prescribe the most effective, efficacious (real-world) medication for the specific disorder. Overall, an approach of carefully considered individual prescribing is recommended. One important element of this is to consider the potential negative impact of medication side effects on athletic performance. This is accompanied by the need to understand the impact of an athlete's physiologic stresses on both pharmacodynamics and pharmacokinetics (how the athlete's body handles the drug). For example, in the treatment of depression, some Sport Psychiatrists start with bupropion or a selective serotonin reuptake inhibitor (SSRI). The SSRIs usually are the first-line medication for anxiety disorders and posttraumatic stress disorder. Buspirone may help with generalized anxiety disorder and is well tolerated. To treat psychosis, usually schizophrenia, which can affect cognition and function, including playing a sport, the clinician must individualize care based on the clinical presentation as well as using the most effective medication so the athlete can compete—these are risperidone, olanzapine, and, if response is inadequate, clozapine. Some Sports Psychiatrists recommend other antipsychotic medication due to side effects with these 3 medications. The same general approach is true for bipolar disorder and is related to efficacy, safety, side effects, and tolerability.[15] Lithium may be used for bipolar disorders, but fluid changes and drug interactions need to be monitored closely, especially for athletes who lose body water through training and take nonsteroidal anti-inflammatory medications. Medications, such as the sedative-hypnotics/benzodiazepines, all have the potential for abuse and addiction but also can cause psychomotor impairment that can hinder performance. For the treatment of attention-deficit/hyperactivity disorder, because atomoxetine takes longer to work than methylphenidate or amphetamines, many Sport Psychiatrist use the stimulants. Athletes may experience side effects with atomoxetine and it is less potent than the stimulants. If an athlete is on a stimulant and it is working well, there may not be a need to make a change in medication if they are monitored closely. Concern rests with the stimulant about performance enhancement and misuse. Additionally, timing of dose may be important because stimulants may interfere with appetite, weight management and sleep. Thermoregulation, heat injuries, and rhabdomyolysis are factors that should not be overlooked. Therapeutic use exemptions (TUEs) may need to be completed as well.

Athletes who take psychotropic medication should have routine monitoring of weight, vital signs, sleep, energy, and body mass index/lean mass. In addition, depending on the psychotropic medication used, blood work should be followed routinely. This may include complete blood cell count with differential, comprehensive metabolic panel, thyroid studies, electrocardiogram, and lipid panel and possibly a hemoglobin A_{1C}. Monitoring symptoms of an athlete's psychiatric disorder and functional status is important. Performance progression through a tracking process is suggested.

Finally, the Sport Psychiatrist should be familiar with antidoping guidelines and the World Anti-Doping Agency (WADA),[16] WADA Code and Prohibited list of medications and methods in and out of competition and NCAA guidelines before prescribing medication to athletes. The use of TUEs can be used when clinically indicated for some medications.

THE SPORT PSYCHIATRY DOMAIN: OTHER INTERVENTION STRATEGIES USED WITH ATHLETES

With psychological and psychiatric skills increasingly used to support athletes in sport for performance enhancement, there also is a need to evaluate and utilize evidence-based interventions. Several intervention strategies from research have been studied, such as mental practice, goal setting, team building, self-talk, stress management, mental toughness and resilience, and so forth. In addition, there is significant need to develop and implement well-designed intervention studies that target improvement of postinjury psychological outcomes in order to assist injured athletes' successfully recovery from sport injury. Other psychological techniques, such as micro-counseling skills, ACT, and written disclosure, have demonstrated effectiveness in reducing negative psychological consequences, improving psychological coping, and reducing reinjury anxiety. From a Sport Psychiatry perspective, some key areas within the sport domain are discussed briefly utilizing questions and **Box 2** and **Table 1**:

WHERE ARE PSYCHOLOGICAL INTERVENTIONS DELIVERED?
Sports

In the domain of sports, the 2 most common settings for the delivery of psychological interventions are training and competition. Although athletes also use psychological skills in their lives outside of sport, it is common practice that they are delivered in the sport context. This usually is done before or after training at the training venue when working with a team or individual sport athlete. Alternatively, when an athlete or parent seeks out individual consultation, these consultations normally take place at a Sport Psychiatrist's office or a primary care facility.

Exercise

In the context of exercise, psychological interventions are administered most in con-sultations that normally take place at a Sport Psychiatrist's office or at a primary care facility and/or as part of telehealth interventions.

Injury Rehabilitation

Athletes recovering from an injury may use psychological interventions to prevent future injuries, deal with a present injury, or as part of a return-to-play protocol. For example, teaching an injured athlete how to set goals during their rehabilitation pro-cess help them structure their rehabilitation training in small chunks, which aids them in building back their self-confidence and motivation. Teaching the athletes

---

Box 2
Psychological intervention strategies in sport

The Sport Psychiatrist assists athletes in the following areas:
Confidence
Self-regulation and emotional control
Rest and recovery
Attentional control
Resilience to help with setbacks and obstacles (eg, injury and anxiety)

Table 1
What are the outcomes for psychological skills training program?

Confidence	Self-belief and belief in training plans
Concentration	Focus on process and on the present
Imagery	Visualize positive shots, plays, and strategies
Arousal and emotional regulation	Mental and emotional flexibility in different situations
Motivation	Ability to set the process/outcome to overcome barriers
Composure	Ability to relax and find the individualized zone of optimal performance
Resilience	Ability to bounce back emotionally from setbacks/losses
Mental toughness	Learn to develop emotional strength and character to achieve their goals

how to utilize diaphragmatic breathing effectively either with or without biofeedback can ensure they are engaged in the appropriate intensity of exercise can teach athletes to self-regulate their emotions and levels of arousal.

HOW ARE PSYCHOLOGICAL AND PSYCHIATRIC INTERVENTIONS IN ELITE SPORTS DELIVERED?

Although psychological interventions are delivered in a variety of ways, a common approach involves the following phases:

1. Assessment: in the early stage of working with an individual or a team it always is a good idea to assess the athletes on their use of mental skills and or their awareness of what they are doing versus what is happening in competition. An excellent reference on assessment of applied psychological skills in sports can be found in the book edited by Taylor published by Human Kinetics in 2018.[17]
2. Education: in the education phase, athletes learn to recognize what are the basic psychological skills and how these skills have an impact on sport performance and enhance mental toughness. Mental toughness is the ability to consistently perform toward the upper range of talent and skill regardless of competitive circumstances and comprises both resilience and psychological skills (self-belief, focus, and motivation). Mental toughness is a teachable multidimensional skill and has 4 components: (1) attitude/mindset, (2) training, (3) competition, and (4) postcompetition. Mental toughness characteristics include having unshakeable self-belief, coping effectively with pressure and adversity, being resilient (overcome obstacles and failure), thriving on pressure, emotional intelligence (self-awareness, coachability, and emotional control), being committed, and displaying superior focusing skills. Emotional attributes of mental toughness include emotional flexibility and responsiveness, staying emotionally strong under pressure, and being able to bounce back and adapt under pressure.
3. Training: psychological skills generally are taught and implemented and refined in training before utilizing them in competition. This process allows athletes time to individualize these skills within their competition routines. Athletes gain confidence in the process when they see improvement.
4. Simulation: as part of the training process, competition simulation is organized to make training as close to the pressure conditions of competition to examine the efficacy of integrating psychological skills in a performance environment.

5. Evaluation: the last phase of the intervention practice is tracking and monitoring athlete performance throughout the varying phases of competition to evaluate the strengths and areas of improvement of sport performance (eg, reaction-time during start phase for a track athlete).

WHERE AND HOW CAN SPORT PSYCHIATRISTS ENHANCE THEIR COMPETENCIES IN SPORT?

Sport Psychiatrists need to have a good understanding and how to use of psychological or mental skills and how to integrate them within the sports yearly training plan. Gaining understanding of mental skills often requires additional training and the use of mentor to acquire the requisite skills. At face value, terms like composure, attention and concentration, confidence, and commitment appear simple and obvious. After a more detailed investigation and understanding, however, the Sports Psychiatrist can appreciate the depth and use of various constructs that help build psychological skills and strategies for athletes. Examples include the following:

Use of foundation skills to improve goal setting, self-confidence, and commitment

Use of psychosomatic skills to improve fear control, relaxation, activation, stress reactions

Use of cognitive skills for focusing, refocusing, mental rehearsal-imagery/visualization, competition planning, and evaluation

SUMMARY

Challenges for the field include addressing the stigma of mental illness and substance use disorders and providing education so that athletes do not feel that they will be labeled as "crazy" or an "addict" and not allowed to participate. The tendency to idealize athletes can lead the athletic community to deny the exitance of a substance use disorder or other psychiatric disorders. The education of the athletic community by psychiatrists to help create an understanding of mental illness and substance use disorders as well as the value of the subspecialty of Sport Psychiatry to assist with treatment and continued participation is of upmost importance. Another challenge for Sport Psychiatrists is to uphold the ethical standards to avoid treatment with banned substances, such as anabolic steroids, stimulants, or other performance enhancing substances or methods. Expansion of research in the field will be an area where Sport Psychiatrists can play a role, including epidemiology, response to medications, and other treatment modalities and effects on performance. Additional recent challenges include addressing the racial and social injustice that is tied to with access and proper treatment of athletes. Furthermore, understanding and treating athletes that are a part of the LGBTQ+ community will be important. The field is growing and gaining recognition as the broad and deep skills of a Sport Psychiatrist are proving increasing useful in the global world of sports.

Finally, this article describes the field of Sport Psychiatry and the evolving role of a Sport Psychiatrist.[18] The mental health needs of athletes continue to grow and their needs increasingly recognized. Sport Psychiatrist are physicians who have expertise and experience in the pathophysiology, diagnosis, and management of psychiatric illness, including substance use disorders. The Sport Psychiatrist needs to have an understanding of the roles, responsibilities, and interventions of individuals who work with athletes to provide the optimal care and promote safe performance and competition. The tool bag of the Sport Psychiatrist includes a range of psychotherapies, pharmacotherapies, and psychological skills training. The Sport Psychiatrist must be able to design a treatment plan or intervention, communicate with members of the integrated treatment team, and deliver that treatment as indicated, case-by-case.

CLINICS CARE POINTS

- To optimize the diagnostic evaluation and treatment plan, the Sport Psychiatrist should attempt to obtain input from members of the integrated sports team.
- Validated screening tools to identify potential psychiatric and substance problems should be routinely used.
- Measuring and recording progress with treatment can be helpful to monitor progress and in making decisions related to return to practice/play.
- When prescribing psychotropic medication to athletes several factors must be considered including safety, performance, and side effects.
- Be familiar with which medications may require a Therapeutic Use Exemption (TUE) and use the published information from the World Antidoping Agency (WADA) to be aware of prohibited substance and methods for in and out of competition.

REFERENCES

1. Brown GT, Hailine B, Kroshus E, et al. Mind, body and sport understanding and supporting student athlete mental wellness. Indianapolis, IN: National Collegiate Athletic Association; 2014.
2. National Collegiate Athletic Association Sport Science Institute. National Collegiate Athletic Association; Indianapolis, IN: 2016, revised 2020. Mental health best practices: inter-association consensus document: best practices for understanding and supporting student-athlete mental wellness.
3. Bhugra D, Chisolm M, Glick I, et al. International Review of psychiatry. Abingdon, Oxon: Sports Psychiatry; 2016. A Developing field.
4. Reardon DL, Hainline B, Aron CM, et al. Mental health in elite athletes: International Olympic Committee census state. Br J Sports Med 2019;53:667–99.
5. Glick I, Kamis D, Stull T. The ISSP Manual of Sports Psychiatry, 2018.
6. Beisser A. The madness in sports. New York: Appleton-Century-Crofts; 1967.
7. Massamino JH. Sports psychiatry. Ann Sports Med 1987;3:55–8.
8. Begel D, Burton R. Sports Psychiatry. 2000.
9. Schaal K, Tafflet M, Nassif H, et al. Psychological balance in high level athletes: gender-based differences and sport-specific patterns. PLoS One 2011;6(5):e19007.
10. Hausenblas H, Symons Downs D. Comparison of body image between athletes and non athletes review. J Appl Sport Psychol 2001;13(3):323–39.
11. McDuff ER, Garvin M. Working with sports organizations and teams. Int Rev Psychiatry 2016;28:595–605.
12. Currie A, Johnston A. Psychiatric disorders: The psychiatrist's contribution to sport. Int Rev Psychiatry 2016;28:587–94.
13. Butler AC, Chapman JE, Forman EM, et al. The empirical status of cognitive-behavioral therapy: a review of meta-analyses. Clin Psychol Rev 2006 Jan;26(1):17–31.
14. Puig J, Pummell B. "I can't lose this match": CBT and the sports psychologist. Sports Exerc Psychol Rev 2012;8:2.
15. Currie A, Gorczynski P, Rice SM, et al. Bipolar and psychotic disorders in elite athletes: a narrative review. Br J Sports Med 2019;0:1–9.
16. The World Anti-Doping Code International Standard Prohibited List January 2020.
17. Taylor J, editor. Assessment in applied sport psychology. Champaign, IL: Human Kinetics; 2018.
18. Glick I, Reardon C, Stull T. Sports Psychiatry: An Update and the Emerging Role of the Sports Psychiatrist on the Sports Medicine Team. Clin J Sport Med 2020;00:1–2.

Achieving Mental Health and Peak Performance in Elite Athletes

Pierre Beauchamp, PhD[a,1], Danielle Kamis, MD[b,2],
Todd Stull, MD[c,*]

KEYWORDS

- Barriers • Harassment • Stigma • Psychological interventions • Peak performance
- Psychological skills

KEY POINTS

- To optimize performance with athletes, mental health needs must be addressed to achieve peak performance within a high-performance culture.
- Barriers to peak performance include obstacles related to mental health, such as stigma, harassment, abuse, discrimination and other factors impacting life balance.
- The best psychological interventions are carefully planned to address the specific individual needs of athletes at the right time, in the right place and with the right person.
- An intervention plan is recommended to equip leaders in sports to better recognize and respond to the mental health needs of elite athletes.
- Understanding and addressing the influence of social media on performance to create a healthy environment is an ongoing process.
- Peak performance, the superior use of human potential, can be enhanced by initiating a Psychological Skill Training program, which can enhance clutch performance, improve coping with anxiety, and cement an unshakeable self-belief in one's athletic prowess.

INTRODUCTION

A holistic approach is needed for athletes to perform at their best; an approach that requires education and the ability to adapt to stress and pressure within a high-performance environment. Unmanaged stress levels can lead to mental and physical problems that may impair balance in the athlete's life. Stress levels, if severe enough, interfere with energy and recovery, and thus performance. If mental/emotional

[a] Pro Hockey Analytics; [b] Department of Psychiatry and Behavioral Sciences, Stanford University School of Medicine, 401 Quarry Road, Stanford, CA, 94305, USA; [c] Department of Psychiatry and Neuroscience, University of California, Riverside School of Medicine, UCR Health-Citrus Tower, 3390 University Avenue Suite 115, Riverside, CA, 92501, USA
[1] Present address: 254 Waldon Drive, Burlington, Ontario L7N 2A6, Canada.
[2] Present address: 164 Main Street Sui 201, Los Altos, CA 94022.
* Corresponding author.
E-mail address: Todd.stull@ucr.edu

Psychiatr Clin N Am 44 (2021) 347–358
https://doi.org/10.1016/j.psc.2021.04.002
0193-953X/21/© 2021 Elsevier Inc. All rights reserved.

psych.theclinics.com

symptoms become prolonged and severe, an athlete may develop a mental illness. Both genetic and environmental influences play a role in the development of a psychiatric disorder or substance use disorder.

Psychiatric disorders in athletes include adjustment disorders, mood disorders, anxiety and related disorders, sleep disorders, attention deficit hyperactivity disorder, eating disorders and substance use disorders. The first part of this article is focused on social, emotional, physical, and cultural influences that affect performance. It also addresses untreated mental health or substance use disorders, which compromise and limit athletic performance, and in some cases, can be career ending. The second part of the article discusses peak performance, psychological states, psychological skills, mental toughness, and resilience.

LIFE BALANCE IN THE DOMAIN OF THE ATHLETE: SOCIAL, EMOTIONAL, PHYSICAL, AND CULTURAL

Sport is a microcosm of our world, and athletes require tailored mental health treatment. Challenges that stewards of athletic activity face include the following: How well we treat those requiring psychiatric care; how we refrain from senseless harassment, and how we treat treatment of minorities with respect; how we adapt to modern communication; and how we build a supportive team environment and achieve athletic success are all.

Stigma of Mental Health in Sports Remains a Disturbing Opponent

Pervading our culture is a stigma attached to those seeking help with their mental situation. That stigma is prominently present in the minds of athletes.[1] The public frequently sees the world of athletics as a place in which the talented and resilient compete, not a world where the participants require mental health support. Too often, athletes believe that needing or requesting mental health support is associated with weakness; the exact opposite of what athletes want to project and internalize.

There are many factors that incentivize athletes to turn away from psychiatric resources. The most powerful factor is often social stigma, which negatively affects student athletes who have been taught to be tough, push hard, and persist. At certain times, athletes who have been referred for counseling and are in need of therapy may be uncertain why they are being referred in the first place. Their list of rationalizations for avoiding therapy is long but the most powerful factor is often stigma. Athletes may have strong bodies and great endurance; however, athletes experience depression at the same rate as their nonathlete peers. In fact, in some sports, such as track and field, male and female athletes have even higher levels of depression than their nonathletic counterparts.[2] Although the need is there, the stigma of mental health counseling deters athletes from seeking help from therapists and coaches. The athlete's aversion to seeking mental health support is a risk that needs to be recognized and corrected.

In addition to the issue of stigma, athletes worry that if they attend one session, they may be trapped into continuing and ongoing treatment. Many athletes are more interested in the "quick fix" than in the work needed to address underlying issues. In addition, a legitimate obstacle to psychiatric care is the issue of time. High-level athletes and student athletes are under severe time restraints due to a combination of their rigorous training schedules, academic obligations, and work to support their athletic career.

Harassment and Discrimination Toward Minorities

Minority athletes arrive on campus with a set of experiences that may be significantly different from others. In supporting a successful career for minority athletes, a concerted effort by players and coaches must be made to gain an appreciation of the minority athlete's perceptions and experiences.[3] Having insight into a minority's background and upbringing is critical to effectively communicate. For example, the black athlete may have been stopped and frisked due to racial profiling and as a result may feel pressure to appear nonthreatening for fear of being harassed by police. Or, when an athlete from a distinct background arrives on campus, they may feel isolated from the majority.

In addition, athletes may have experienced family violence and in too many cases, they have grown up in single-parent households. A young athlete from a disadvantaged background may have a family that pressures them to succeed; if the athlete is underperforming or loses interest in sports, there may be a strong pushback from those who have sacrificed for their athletic career. Serious consequences can occur when the athlete underperforms or loses interest in sport. The family may feel cheated and lay a burden on the athlete. Many adolescent athletes burn out and abandon sports, a fact true for both minority and nonminority athletes.

To effectively address the needs of the minority athlete, an integrative outreach program needs to be put into action from the beginning. Within this outreach program, mental health supports with an understanding of the athlete's background, history, and needs will proactively help provide for mental and thus performance success.

Harassment and Discrimination Toward Lesbian, Gay, Bisexual, Transgender, Queer or Questioning Students

A societal change has taken place in the LGBTQ (Lesbian, Gay, Bisexual, Transgender, Queer or Questioning) community. Historically, many students arrived on college campuses without feeling safe to overtly express their sexual orientation. Now, it is common for the LGBTQ student to arrive on campus with sexual orientation already expressed.[3] Despite cultural changes, some coaches, administrators, and student athletes continue to exhibit heterosexist and homophobic attitudes.

At times, some heterosexual student athletes are in denial that team members are part of the LGBTQ community and even express negative reactions to their teammate. This burden of discrimination appears to be a contributing factor to the elevated incidence of depression, alcohol and drug abuse, and suicide attempts in these individuals. Harassment of the LGBTQ community needs to be confronted. Negative language leveled against LGBTQ athletes must be prohibited and this prohibition should be extended to fans. Comprehensive mental health counseling with the intent of equal treatment as well as deeper insights into the discrimination faced by LGBTQ athletes is vital to support this group of athletes.

Additional Elements of Stress in the Athletic Environment

Athletes experience extreme stress from time demands, coaching pressures, and interactions with their environment, which may overwhelm the athlete and discourage them from seeking mental health therapy. Stress is not inherently negative if it is managed and controlled, and even can promote growth. However, if stress is not properly addressed, it can result in negative health outcomes either directly or through unhealthy coping measures such as substance abuse. When thinking about National Collegiate Athletic Association athletes who are subjected to enormous time demands and stresses, a discord exists. Many college athletes know that their future does not involve professional sports. In addition, many student athletes, with goals of developing a professional career outside of sport, have the desire to graduate with good grades. Although at the same time, after practicing for 30 hours a week, and spending a whole day traveling for a game, a football player may be under terrible stress knowing that there is difficult math midterm the day after returning to campus. The balance among sports, academics, and engaging in the college experience can lead to internal turmoil and distress.

Another frequent source of stress is the internal pressure to compete successfully compounded by external pressures from coaches, parents, and friends. The coach's own evaluation and compensation may hinge on the competitive results of the student athlete. This pressure, in turn, may be transferred onto the athlete contributing to greater anxiety and distress. If athletes have poor communication with their coaches, they are at risk for negative mental health outcomes such as depression, burnout, and sleep disorders. If teammates and coaches stigmatize mental health or encourage a culture of toughness at all costs, symptomatic or at-risk individuals will be less likely to disclose their mental health needs.

Although the athletic environment presents many risk factors for an athlete's mental health, it can also be a source for support for wellness and success. Diminishing sources of stress, removing the mental health stigma, providing first class mental health resources, and encouraging those in need to seek mental health assistance can improve the well-being of the student athlete.

The Athletic World Can Create Vulnerabilities for Abuse

It has been reported that most perpetrators of abuse originated from coaches, teachers, and instructors who were male and ranged in age from 16 to 63 years old.[4] In a consensus statement, the International Olympic Committee Athlete Commission reported sexual harassment ranging upward to 92% and sexual abuse ranging upward to 49%. The data here are startling. Available information suggests that most victims were young females but a significant underreporting by male victims is suspected.[4]

The first step in aiding athletes, especially those who are underage who have experienced abuse, is open communication with their parents. Parents should establish a mature open relationship with both of their female and children. No questions or details about physical contact are off limits. Parents should feel comfortable checking in with their child athlete. If a parent or child reports abuse to a pediatrician, state law, in all 50 states, requires the physician to report these concerns.

Second, colleges should provide all collegiate athletes with the name of a specific college official to report any alleged abuse. That specific point person should meet with all female and male athletes early in the year to introduce themselves and establish an open line of communication as well as create an environment in which athletes can be confident that they are protected.

The Importance of Social Media to the Athlete

Social media has revolutionized the way we interact and the way we communicate, and its influence will continue to grow. It is widely believed that if you are not interacting, generating, or consuming information, you are behind the times. Athletes should understand the importance of social media and how it may be critical to their future. The large advantage of athletes using social networking is to make career connections, network, and become known. Social networking can help athletes get recruited as well as establish important contacts.

There is also a downside to social networking that athletes must understand to avoid harming their future. Many athletes admit to posting something inappropriate on their social media accounts: For example, a Philadelphia professional athlete posted an inappropriate reference to Hitler that led to a backlash from sportswriters and fans. If an athlete posts something embarrassing or critical of another group, they may pay major consequences. Another important note is that once information is disseminated, it cannot be taken back. With these real dangers, it is key for athletes to learn about ethics and guidelines before posting information. On a parallel note, adolescents and college athletes should be encouraged to spend time with one another outside their sport so they can explore other interests in-person instead of relying on social media as their social outlet.

How to Create a Wholesome Climate for Athletes

Although athletes spend most of their time training and competing, there are other aspects of their life that contribute to a healthier life balance. Coaches and parents must recognize the athlete's allegiance to the team, which may at times may be given priority over the allegiance to the parent or coach. Efforts should be made to foster a safe environment in which athletes spend time together and speak openly to one another. It can be critical to promote an environment that exalts team accomplishments rather than individual success. On a team, an environment that promotes constructive feedback should be cultivated towards psychological safety. For example, after a game, the athletes might sit in a circle. Each athlete can be given the chance to express something positive about their teammate and something they could improve on. Creating this expected routine can help build togetherness and cut down on behind-the-back negative comments.

Athletes and the Need for Supportive Help from Friends and Family: No Man Is an Island

Certainly, a high level of confidence and belief in one's own athletic ability affects success, but having a support system of friends and family, and backed up by a strong team can be just as important. According to Professor Tim Rees, in some cases, it appears that this support team is the single most important factor in athletic success.[5] The encouragement and support from friends and family can lead to confidence to compete successfully in high-pressure athletic competition.

Conclusion

There are multiple factors that affect the mental well-being of athletes. These factors include having a social support network composed of friends, family, coaches, trainers, and access to mental health support. In addition, creating a safe environment in which athletes are not discriminated against is essential. Athletes need to be allowed to feel comfortable discussing vulnerabilities with therapists. It is crucial that athletes have access to a safe training environment in which harassment is forbidden. Last, athletes must be educated on social media presence including awareness that the way in which they depict themselves in social media can have a large impact on their athletic career.

PEAK PERFORMANCE WITHIN A HIGH-PERFORMANCE CULTURE
What Is a High-Performance Culture in Sport?

Citius, Altius, Fortius, or "Faster, Higher, Stronger" slogan is based on the highly ideological concept of Olympic sport and framed by the idea that winning an Olympic gold medal is the pinnacle of sport achievement. Due to the globalization of sports and the unique nature of the Olympic Games, this magnitude brings with it enormous pressure on sport organizations and athletes to perform for their country. From a performance enhancement perspective, the notion that the organizational culture plays a key function on the impact of athlete performance is a relatively new and emerging topic in applied sport science and psychology literature.[6]

In business, organizational effectiveness that drives a high-performance work culture is an organization that achieves better financial and nonfinancial results than those of its peers over a long period of time. Organizational change in this way requires many skills such as adaptive leadership in which people are mobilized to tackle tough challenges and thrive.[7] Norms for high-performance culture may differ regionally and between various sports. Applied work in Sport Psychology and Psychiatry is generally focused on intra-individual and team perspectives; however, little or no attention has been given as to whether an optimal climate exists for the development of athletes. Consequently, development of high-performance culture with good mental health is an emerging focus in Sport Psychology/Psychiatry intervention research.[8]

One example of creating a high-performance culture is through the concept known as "marginal gains," an approach to performance improvement in elite sports that came from British Cycling during the London 2012 Olympic Games where British Cycling won a total of 8 gold medals. At the time, British cyclists had only won 1 gold medal since 1908. Dave Brailsford was hired as the High-Performance Director of Team GB to put the team on a new trajectory. What made his leadership style different was his relentless commitment to a strategy referred to as "the aggregation of marginal gains," which was the philosophy of breaking down every component of a bike race into its individual components and then improving it by 1% to get a cumulative increase in performance. The components include everything from hand washing to training hours to nutrition and sleep quality to technology and leadership. This transformational leadership impacts everything from organizational vision and mindset, coaching leadership, to the athletes' motivational engagement. However, recent accounts and awareness among Team GB athletes have demonstrated this pressurized environment to succeed may well make athletes more vulnerable to poor mental health, which can in turn reduce the likelihood of them seeking help when it is most needed.

Peak Performance in Sports

Peak performance occurs when an athlete experiences a strong sense of self-belief and performs up to (and sometimes exceeds) their full potential.[9] While having a peak performance, athletes are more efficient, creative and rely on automaticity to achieve their goals due to heightened optimal functioning. The search for what constitutes the ideal psychological state to gain peak performance, and what factors play a role, have been prominent areas of study in sport psychology research.

Psychological States and Optimal Functioning in Sport

Peak performance describes an athlete performing at their optimum level of functioning in competition and producing outstanding results. It is associated theoretically with automatic functioning at the upper limits of performance, usually involving self-regulation of factors relevant to their environment and is related to a state of accomplishment that comes as a consequence of sustained effort and concentration, see **Box 1**.

A clutch response is "any performance increment or superior performance that occurs under pressure circumstances."[11] The term "clutch" performance originated from statistical analysis of hitting in the baseball postseason. Recently, studies on the psychological states underlying peak performance termed "clutch performance under pressure" such as winning a golf tournament found improved performance under pressure was characterized by clutch states that included heightened and deliberate concentration, intense effort and heightened awareness under the purposeful, effortful, and intense state described as "making it happen" versus "letting it happen."[12]

Furthermore, athletes who use approach-based coping strategies such as pre-shot and post-shot routines (external focus on task-oriented cues), reappraising

---

Box 1
Psychological profile associated with peak performance[10]

- Self-confidence
- Expectations of success
- Energized but relaxed
- Feeling in control
- High level of focus on the task
- Positive attitudes and thoughts about performance
- Determined and fully committed

---

threatening stressors (lowering expectations), and placing oneself under pressure during practice to rehearse coping strategies (greater focus on self-improvement) have been found to be more successful under pressure versus those who choked and vented their frustrations and emotions.[13] These findings provide evidence that clutch performance under pressure is a skill that coaches and Sport Psychologists/Psychiatrists can teach athletes to perform.

Psychological Skills Training for Peak Performance in Sport

The effectiveness of psychological skills training (PST) on performance has been well established. Vealey,[14] in a review of PST programs, suggested 3 areas for the development of PST interventions: (1) the need for sport-specific PST programs whereby psychological practice was incorporated with physical training; (2) emphasis on teaching athletes how to set individualized competition plans for their sport; and (3) the need for a process approach within the PST program. In addition, many applied consultants in the field suggest that packaging or grouping of psychological strategies into a program approach can be effective when working with individual and or team sports, see **Box 2**.[15]

The integration of a successful PST program approach requires a combination of psychological skills training with the specific needs of the athlete. Factors taken into consideration include age, gender, years and level of experience, the specific

---

Box 2
An applied Olympic Psychological Skills Training integrative approach to performance under pressure[7]

1. Understanding anxiety and learning to use breathing skills as an ally to balance the autonomic nervous system
2. Reframing internal language to reappraise feelings about pressure and external body language to boost self-confidence
3. Learning to use self-referenced norms for improvement and focus on the task versus the ego of winning
4. Understanding life balance and having perspective on what is really important in life
5. Fully committing with self-belief in the process of training and competing within the team context
6. Mental rehearsal for the big day, possibly using simulation training to see and feel yourself being on the big stage performing your best and besting personal or World Records
7. Sensory shutdown within the pre-competition routine to narrow attention

demands of the sport (technical, tactical, physical, and mental), and the environmental demands of the sport. Previous research in the area of periodization training leading to elite athletic performance through the utilization of quadrennial and yearly training plans (YTP) has made a significant contribution to the art and science of YTPs. Recently, researchers have proposed an integrated periodized PST program over consecutive training cycles whereby education, skill acquisition, and implementation of skills allow for long-term development while directly reflecting individual needs and differences.[16]

Finally, from a professional practice perspective, the ultimate goal of all PST programs is to render the athletes autonomous and effectively functioning on their own without the direction of the coach or Sport Psychology/Psychiatry consultant. Consequently, the athlete should be able to self-regulate their internal functioning in the face of competitive and noncompetitive environmental demands while allowing the Sport Psychology/Psychiatry consultant to "fade out" as the athlete approaches major competitions. Furthermore, research has supported Kirschenbaum's[17] self-regulation model in sports when dealing with environmental demands.

Mental Toughness in Sport

Coaches and athletes contribute toward the environmental process of cultivating mental toughness (MT) by their actions and behaviors within their sport-specific culture. MT is multidimensional in scope and related to successful performance and outcomes.[18] Attributes most often reported to represent MT include having unshakeable self-belief, coping effectively with pressure and adversity, being resilient, thriving on pressure, being committed, and displaying superior focusing and refocusing skills when distracted. Jones and colleagues[19] contextualized MT into 4 dimensions:

1. Attitude/Mindset (a mentally tough performer has cultivated an exceptional ability to focus, and exhibits strong self-belief in their sport abilities)
2. Training (a mentally tough performer embraces the difficult aspects of training and can "produce the quality" in even the most mundane workouts)
3. Competition (a mentally tough performer thrives under pressure, rising to the top when pressure is highest)
4. Post-Competition (a mentally tough performer makes attributions for success and failure that allow them to continue to compete with confidence in the present moment)

MT is a long-term and complex process that is influenced by the athlete's personal qualities, the sport environment, and critical incidents that define the actions of both athletes and coaches.[20] It is the state of being more consistent and better than your opponents by matching your intensity with theirs and by being more determined, focused, confident, and in control emotionally under pressure. To develop this psychological edge, applied intervention focuses on 3 attributes:

1. Psychological skills to enhance MT (eg, self-belief, focus, motivation)
2. Emotional intelligence: awareness of emotional self-regulation (for example, coachability, control of training environment, push themselves beyond physical limits, maintain control on poor training days, pressure regulation, handle failure and success appropriately)
3. Resilience or coping skills to overcome obstacles and setbacks (eg, dealing with failure, overcoming obstacles in training and life, injuries).

A multidimensional strategy is used before, during, and after events to build and maintain MT, see **Box 3**.

Box 3
A multidimensional strategy to build or maintain mental toughness

1. Use mental toughness game plans for success (week and night before plans, pre-competition plans, competition game plans, and post-competition debriefs)

2. Model and recalling previous successful events (daily imagery or mental rehearsal and/or self-hypnosis can help athletes feel more confident in their performance preparation) and readiness for competition

3. Initiate active and passive recovery techniques (eg, stretching, hydrotherapy, cryotherapy, nutrition, massage and myofascial release, compression therapy, sleep, naps and sleep deprivation, red and near-infrared light therapy, intermittent hypoxia training, heart rate variability breathing)

4. Implement athlete management systems (eg, athlete monitoring of data: daily wellness indicators, external load parameters, internal load physiologic parameters, weekly functional tests data, medical data, and biomarker data)

5. Periodization of training and competition (eg, 4-year quadrennial plans, annual training plans, Olympic year training and competition plans, tapering and peaking in individual and team sports)

Resilience in Sports

The American Psychological Association defines psychological resilience as "the process of adapting well in the face of adversity, trauma, tragedy, threats or significant sources of stress."[21] Investigating the relationship between peak performance and psychological resilience after the London 2012 Olympic Games, researchers interviewed 12 Olympic Gold medalists and developed the Grounded Theory of Psychological Resilience of Olympic Champions.[22] Their findings identified positive personality, motivation, confidence, focus, and perceived social support as the key factors related to resilience. These factors protected the world's best athletes from the potential negative effect of stressors by influencing their challenge appraisal and meta-cognitions.[23] These constructive cognitive reactions help create advantageous responses that may lead to Olympic peak performances.

From a team perspective, resilience has been defined as a "dynamic psychosocial process which protects a group of individuals from the potential negative effect of the stressors they collectively encounter - comprises of the processes whereby team members use their individual and collective resources to positively adapt when experiencing adversity."[24] Research on a World Cup–winning rugby team has revealed 5 main psychosocial processes underlying team resilience: (1) transformational leadership, (2) shared team leadership, (3) team learning, (4) team identity, and (5) positive emotions. In this team context, rugby players appraised stressors from a positive perspective and the focus was on moving forward as a team despite setbacks. It is also import to recognize that athletes operate within organizational climates that have imbedded cultural and similar sport-specific influences that would negate the impact of "canned" resilience interventions that would be effective across all athletes, teams and sport organizations. Buy-in from all stakeholders that consider the sport culture is critical before embarking on a team-wide resilience intervention. Moreover, beyond sports, resilience intervention needs to also consider issues related to mental health, disadvantaged individuals and minority groups.

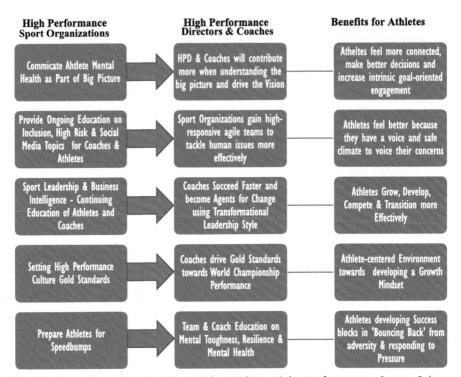

Fig. 1. Integration of Mental Health Within High Performance Sport Culture Recommendations.

Organizational Dynamics Related to Mental Toughness and Resilience

An organization's capacity for resilience and development of MT can be cultivated via environmental influences within the sport organization; it can be assessed and taught through the integration of both mental skills and resilience training programs.[25] Examples include (1) developing an organizational capacity for resilience (eg, strong core values, sense of purpose and identity); (2) high-performance directors and coach education (eg, transformational leadership, shared team leadership and agile decision-making); (3) mental skills and mental health training for athletes (eg, MT, resilience, emotional regulation, mindfulness); (4) sport organizations creating a healthy, enjoyable, competitive motivational climate (eg, safe and supportive social networks); and (5) providing culturally sensitive resilience training for athletes, coaches, and management (eg, Acceptance and Commitment Therapy).[26] However, the idea that mental health is entirely a person factor neglects to acknowledge the more national systemic problem or the local organizational level: the sources of stress that could and should be addressed systemically to facilitate coping and resilience among all stakeholders. Overall, the convergence of evidence points toward the importance of organizational dynamics within a high-performance culture in sport organizations that would allow athletes to embrace learning from both their success and failures in sport, and also toward awareness of transferable skills and building successful transitions out of sport.

SUMMARY

The athlete's development, peak performance, and mental health and well-being are all integrated from a holistic perspective. Creating and maintaining a high-performance culture on regional, national, and Olympic stages are important contextual components of an integrated training and competition environment. Transformational leadership to take on tough challenges in sports can be achieved to affect organizational systemic change by being adaptive and responsive to the needs of athletes and coaches. Adaptation requires continuous learning. Human performance is a function of many influences on athletes, coaches, and high-performance directors and their organizations. It is a combination of these factors that results in the desired performance and the associated leadership behaviors that support the performance culture. **Fig. 1** provides an integrate holistic and life-span perspective that we believe can positively impact the mental well-being of the athlete, maximize training and readiness for competition, and ultimately facilitate the successful transition for athletes out of their sport careers.

DISCLOSURE

The authors have nothing to disclose.

REFERENCES

1. McLean B. Stigma of mental health in sports remains an opponent. NAMI News 2014. Available at: www.nami.org/About-NAMI/NAMI-News/2014/Stigma-of-Mental-Health-in-Sports-Remains-an-Option.
2. Wolanin A, et al. "Prevalence of clinically elevated depressive symptoms in college athletes and differences by gender and sport," NIH. National Library of Medicine, National Center for Biotechnology Information, Pub Med.Gov; 2016. Available at: pubmed.ncbi.nlm.nih.gov/26782764/.
3. NCAA. "Mind body and sports harassment and discrimination," NCAA, Mind Body Sports Homepage. Available at: http://www.ncaa.org/sport-science-institute/mind-body-and-sport.
4. LaBotz M, et al. Athletic environments can create opportunities for abuse. AAP News 2018. Available at: http://www.aappublications.org/news/2018/02/23/coaches022318#:%7E:%20text=Abuse%20by%20peers%20within%20sporting,for%20abuse%2C%20particularly%20among%20peers. Accessed September 2, 2020.
5. Steffens N, Slade E, Stevens M, et al. Putting the 'we' into workout: The association of identity leadership with exercise class attendance and effort, and the mediating role of group identification and comfort. Psychol Sports Exerc 2019; 45:101544.
6. Henriksen K. Developing a high-performance culture: a sport psychology intervention from an ecological perspective in elite orienteering. J Sport Psychol Action 2015;6(3):141–53.
7. Beauchamp MK, Harvey R, Beauchamp P. An integrated biofeedback and psychological skills training program for canada's olympic short-track speedskating team. J Clin Sport Psychol 2012;6:67–84.
8. Cruickshank A, Collins D. Change management: the case of the elite sport performance team. J Change Manag 2012;12:209–29.
9. Privette G. Peak experience, peak performance, and flow: A comparative analysis of positive human experiences. J Pers Soc Psychol 1983;45:1361–8.
10. Jackson S, Wrigley W. Optimal experience in sport: current issues and future directions. In: Morris T, Summers J, editors. Sport psychology: theories, applications, and issues. 2nd 10 edition. Milton (Queensland): Jacaranda; 2004. p. 423–51.

11. Otten M. Choking vs. clutch performance: a study of sport performance under pressure. J Sport Exerc Psychol 2009;31:583–601.
12. Swann C, Keegan R, Crust L, et al. Psychological states underlying excellent performance in professional golfers: "Letting it happen" vs. "making it happen". Psychol Sport Exerc 2016;23:101–13.
13. Hill D, Hemmings B. A phenomenological exploration of coping responses associated with choking in sport. Qualit Res Sport Exerc Health 2015;23:521–38.
14. Vealey RS. Future directions in psychological skills training. Sport Psychol 1988; 2:318–36.
15. Weinberg RS, Colmar W. The effectiveness of psychological interventions in competitive sport. Sports Med 1994;18:406–18.
16. Lidor R, Blumenstein B, Tenenbaum G. Psychological aspects of training in European basketball: conceptualization, periodization, and planning. Sport Psychol 2007;21:353–67.
17. Kirschenbaum DS. Self-regulation and sport psychology: nurturing an emerging symbiosis. J Sport Psychol 1984;6:159–83.
18. Clough PJ, Earle K, Sewell D. Mental toughness: the concept and its measurement. In: Cockerill I, editor. Solutions in sport psychology. London: Thomson; 2002. p. 32–43.
19. Jones G, Hanton S, Connaughton D. A framework of mental toughness in the world's best performers. Sport Psychol 2007;21:243–64.
20. Connaughton D, Hanton S, Jones G. The development and maintenance of mental toughness in the world's best performers. Sport Psychol 2010;24:168–93.
21. APA. What is resilience. 2012. Available at: www.apa.org/topics/resilience#.
22. Fletcher D, Sarkar M. A grounded theory of psychological resilience in Olympic champions. Psychol Sport Exerc 2012;13:669–78.
23. Sarkar M, Fletcher D. Psychological resilience in sport performers: A review of stressors and protective factors. J Sports Sci 2014;32:1419–34.
24. Morgan PBC, Fletcher D, Sarkar M. Understanding team resilience in the world's best athletes: A case study of a rugby union World Cup winning team. Psychol Sport Exerc 2015;16:91–100.
25. Gucciardi DF, Jackson B, Coulter TJ, et al. The Connor-Davidson Resilience Scale (CD-RISC): dimensionality and age-related measurement invariance with Australian cricketers. Psychol Sport Exerc 2011;12:423–33.
26. Gardner FL, Moore ZE. A mindfulness-acceptance-commitment-based approach to athletic performance enhancement: theoretical considerations. Behav Ther 2004;35:707–23.

Burnout and Motivation in Sport

Paul H. Groenewal, PsyD[a], David Putrino, PT, PhD[b],*, Marissa R. Norman, PsyD[a]

KEYWORDS

- Burnout • Athlete burnout • Motivation • Self-determination theory
- Sports performance

KEY POINTS

- Burnout is the sustained feeling of emotional exhaustion, depersonalization, and inadequate personal accomplishment; within the context of sports, burnout is a state of sport devaluation, physical and emotional exhaustion, and reduced accomplishment.
- Sensitive and specific biomarkers of burnout currently do not exist.
- The clinical gold standards for measuring burnout are the Athlete Burnout Questionnaire and the Maslach Burnout Inventory.
- Motivation models are helpful in preventing and treating burnout.
- Motivational interventions include self-talk, mental imagery, and goal setting.

INTRODUCTION

The investment (both time and money) in sports continues to increase. At the collegiate Division I level, athletes devote on average 34 hours a week to athletics.[1] Many college athletes have reported specializing in their sport before the age of 12 and growing up playing year-round. Concurrently, the importance of Sport Psychology and Psychiatry in supporting the athlete is evolving and highlighting the need for research to expand the understanding of practices/habits/behaviors that impact the athlete's ability to perform.

There is a growing appreciation of burnout and its impact on performance: For individuals, burnout leads to underperformance, compromises physical and psychological well-being, and can lead to a dropout from sports.[2] It negatively impacts an athlete's ability to reach their full potential and can generalize to other areas of life. Burnout also has implications on a team's performance and its cohesiveness. The reported rates of athlete burnout vary in the literature, but overall appears to be in the range of 2% to 11%.[3] This low number may be the result of selection bias and

[a] Inspire Wellness, 266 Harristown Road, Suite 209, Glen Rock, NJ 07452, USA; [b] Department of Rehabilitation and Human Performance, Icahn School of Medicine at Mount Sinai, 1 Gustave L. Levy Pl, Box 1240, New York, NY 10029, USA
* Corresponding author.
E-mail address: david.putrino@mountsinai.org

Psychiatr Clin N Am 44 (2021) 359–372
https://doi.org/10.1016/j.psc.2021.04.008
0193-953X/21/© 2021 Elsevier Inc. All rights reserved.

sampling errors; however, even though burnout appears to impact a small number of athletes, it is reasonable to assume that there is a far-reaching impact on teams and sports in general.

A CONCEPTUAL UNDERSTANDING OF BURNOUT

Although there is considerable talk about burnout within the sports community, researchers are less than exact in terms of defining it, and there is no agreed upon definition of athlete burnout. In order to develop an understanding of burnout, it is helpful to consider the initial conceptualization and how that conceptualization has changed over the years.

Maslach's Initial Conceptualization

Research in burnout began with health care and human service workers. Early theories could be characterized as a psychosocial construct to explain physical and mental deterioration and workplace ineffectiveness. In 1981, this was operationalized when the Maslach Burnout Inventory (MBI) was created and defined burnout using 3 components:[4]

1. Sustained feelings of emotional exhaustion
2. Depersonalization (ie, cynical attitudes and feelings toward their clients)
3. Inadequate personal accomplishments (ie, a sense of low accomplishment and professional inadequacy)

Cognitive-Affect Model of Burnout

One of the earliest models to conceptualize burnout, while also applying the concept to athletes, was proposed by Smith[5] in the cognitive-affective model of athlete burnout. This model is concordant with other models describing burnout as the result of chronic stress but includes physical, mental, and behavioral components. Withdrawal is a prominent feature, including psychological, emotional, and at times physical withdrawal from activities that were previously pursued and enjoyed. Smith used Social Exchange Theory (SET) to differentiate between those who physically withdrew from sports as a result of burnout versus those who withdrew because of other factors. SET postulates that people are motivated by a desire to maximize the positive and minimize the negative. Positive rewards may include tangible items (eg, money, properties, trophies) or psychological ones (eg, goal achievement, feelings of competence, the admiration of others). Negatives, or costs, may include, but are not limited to, the amount of time and effort expended, feelings of failure or the disapproval of others, and/or negative emotions.

Emphasizing the Physical Manifestation of Burnout

Silva[6] examined the impact of physical training on athlete burnout, adding to the discussion of the physical manifestation. This model, focused on the "Training Stress Syndrome," suggests that overtraining in volume and intensity leads to negative adaptation, which in turn may lead to burnout. However, burnout appears to be better explained by chronic exposure to psychosocial stress rather than by the dynamics that explain and lead to overtraining. It does help to increase the focus on the physical aspects of burnout.

Emphasizing the Athlete's Identity and Perceived Control

Coakley[7] proposed that burnout results from social processes, specifically, a lack of opportunity to develop an identity outside of sports and a restricted and demanding environment that limits autonomy and independence. These contributing factors of burnout in athletes leads to stress, which Coakley suggests is directly triggered by burnout rather than the cause of it (unlike the Cognitive-Affective Stress Model). In other words, burnout is a reaction to the exposure of the repressive environment rather than a cause of burnout. Coakley also suggested that burnout created an opportunity to exercise personal autonomy and self beyond a singular athletic identity (in this case, burnout might be good). Coakley's conceptualization of burnout adds value to the exploration of burnout in that it moves the discussion toward a consideration of the sporting environment that is created.

A Model Focused on Athlete Burnout

As seen in **Fig. 1**, Raedeke[8] defines athlete burnout as "a syndrome of physical/emotional exhaustion, sport devaluation and reduced athletic accomplishment." This definition was created by building on existing definitions while tailoring it to better represent the athlete community, and to account for athletes who experience physical and emotional exhaustion as a result of the high demands associated with sport participation rather than simply burning out. Considering this definition, both physical exhaustion and emotional exhaustion are referring to the feeling of fatigue resulting from sport participation. The sport devaluation element of this definition constitutes a lack of meaning or desire experienced by an athlete in their sport and a carelessness regarding their sport performance. The combination of fatigue and the devaluation of sport contributes to the athletes reduced accomplishments.

Raedeke and Smith adjusted the Maslach and Jackson model by adding physical exhaustion to the dimension of exhaustion.[8] This adjustment is important, as athletes are more likely to experience physical fatigue at levels that negatively impact their performance. Second, Raedeke and Smith focused on "sport devaluation" and dropped "depersonalization," meaning that an athlete's job performance is better characterized by their perceived relationship to their sport (ie, a diminished and cynical outlook of the benefits of sport involvement) than by their relationship to others. Although this model seems to ignore the relational elements of sport, it is the current gold standard for conceptualizing athlete burnout.

NEUROBIOLOGY OF BURNOUT

From a physiologic perspective, entering a state of "burnout" is a highly nebulous construct. Literature surrounding the neurobiology of burnout is largely inconclusive

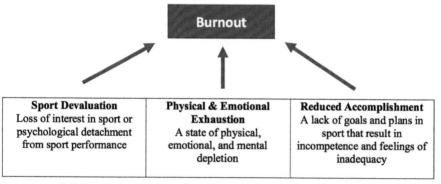

Fig. 1. Item definitions adapted from the ABQ. The 3 main components of athlete burnout include sport devaluation, physical and emotional exhaustion, and reduced sense of accomplishment. (*Data from* Raedeke TD, Smith AL. Development and preliminary validation of an athlete burnout measure. J Sport Exerc Psychol 2001; 23: 281-306.)

and is a reminder that meaningful, objective evaluation of a highly dynamic system, such as the nervous system, is incredibly challenging.

Electroencephalographic Biomarkers of Burnout

Electroencephalography (EEG) is often favored as a human research tool in neuroscience, as it is noninvasive. Interestingly, there are some consistent EEG findings associated with burnout. The most commonly reported finding is a reduction in alpha power during eyes open EEG recording when compared with the controls.[9–11] In addition, certain reductions in the amplitude of quantitative EEG biomarkers are associated with burnout. Individuals who are clinically diagnosed with burnout have also shown a comparative reduction in the amplitude of the P300 event-related potential that occurs in response to an auditory oddball task.[10]

Although these findings are intriguing, it is unclear if there is a practical use of EEG as a biomarker for burnout. EEG measures of burnout do not have an established level of reliability, nor are there meaningful recommendations for specific levels of resting alpha frequency or P300 amplitude that clinicians can use as a diagnostic criterion. In addition, another confounding issue in using EEG as a biomarker of burnout is that EEG findings in individuals who have been clinically diagnosed with burnout and those with depression are highly similar and often indistinguishable.

Although EEG has potential as a biomarker of burnout, currently it does not have the sensitivity to stand alone as a diagnostic criterion. More research is required. In addition, there is little convincing literature to show that burnout interventions can alter the EEG in such a way that they will begin to neurophysiologically resemble a normative population as they begin to recover. The ability to directionally track these biomarkers as they relate to symptom severity is a crucial feature of a trustworthy biomarker and is thus a priority for future EEG research in burnout.

Brain Imaging and Burnout

Functional MRI (fMRI) is an imaging technique that infers neural activity in different regions of the brain based on changes in regional blood flow. Similarly, PET scanning of the brain uses the injection and perfusion of a variety of radioactive tracers to monitor brain metabolism, allowing radiologists to make inferences about brain functioning at rest, during stimulus presentation, or during performance of a cognitive task. Like EEG, fMRI and PET scans are popular methodologies for human neuroscience research because of their minimally invasive nature, and have been used to investigate the neurobiology of burnout.

The link between empathy and burnout is frequently cited in the literature, and therefore, many fMRI studies have focused on investigating the possible relationship between empathy-related regions of the brain and burnout severity. In a study of health care professionals, increased burnout severity was associated with reduced activation of the anterior insular and inferior frontal gyrus.[12] Similarly, in another study of health professionals suffering from burnout, reduced activity in the right dorsolateral prefrontal cortex and middle frontal gyrus was associated with higher levels of self-reported depersonalization, whereas higher reporting of emotional exhaustion was associated with increased activity in the posterior cingulate cortex and middle frontal gyrus.[13] In addition to evidence of burnout causing altered neural activity in higher brain regions associated with empathy, lower limbic areas of the brain have also been shown to exhibit functional changes in imaging studies. For instance, a PET imaging study conducted by Jovanovi and colleagues[14] reported that participants who scored greater than 3.0 on the Maslach Stress-Burnout Inventory-General Survey (MBI-GS) had a significant reduction in functional connectivity between the amygdala and the anterior cingulate gyrus/medial prefrontal cortex compared with a control group that scored less than 3.0 on the MBI-GS. In this cohort, the degree of reported stress was negatively correlated with 5-HT_{1A} receptor binding potential in the amygdala and hippocampus and reduced activity in the anterior cingulate cortex. These findings were replicated in an MRI study, showing that individuals who scored higher than 3.0 on the MBI-GS had significantly weakened functional connectivity between the amygdala and the anterior cingulate cortex when compared with a control cohort that scored less than 3.0 on the MBI-GS.[15] Reduced functional connectivity between the 2 brain regions was correlated with a reduced ability to regulate negative emotion.

In addition to changes in functional connectivity and activation of specific brain regions in participants exhibiting signs and symptoms of burnout, structural changes may also be evident in the brain as a result of burnout. These studies have reported reduced gray matter volume in the anterior cingulate cortex, dorsolateral prefrontal cortex, putamen, and caudate, with gray matter volume in these regions correlating negatively with the degree of stress and increased gray matter volume in the amygdala.[16]

Taken together, the imaging research helps to support the hypothesis that burnout may be a progressive condition, whereby stress-related excitotoxicity results in structural and functional changes in the brain that inevitably lead to impaired cognitive processes and emotion regulation. However, similar to the EEG data presented, the imaging studies cited here show only group effect differences, not a sensitive measure that can be used to diagnose burnout. Thus, given the current state of the science, these methods are research tools in need of further investigation; findings must be taken as part of the larger clinical picture of the athlete rather than a stand-alone diagnostic test.

The Hypothalamus-Pituitary-Adrenal Axis and Burnout

The Hypothalamus-Pituitary-Adrenal axis (HPA axis) is a complex and interconnected neuroendocrine system that is largely responsible for the body's response to stress, as well as many other homeostatic functions. Given the role of the HPA axis in governing acute stress response, it has been a natural topic of burnout-related research for many researchers. Because of its central role in mobilizing physiologic resources during periods of increased metabolic demand, including stress, many studies focus primarily on monitoring cortisol levels as a biomarker of HPA axis function. However, this assumes that burnout is, at its core, simply a condition of chronic stress, when the reality appears to be more complex. The literature surrounding burnout and cortisol levels is inconsistent, with some studies reporting chronically elevated cortisol levels in individuals with burnout in comparison to controls, whereas others have reported no difference, or reduced levels.[17]

With difficulties in establishing a consistent, directional link between cortisol levels and burnout, studies have also begun to investigate other biomarkers that may be analogues of HPA axis dysfunction, such as serum brain-derived neurotrophic factor (sBDNF) levels. BDNF is a crucial component of neuronal survival and neurogenesis in areas of the brain, such as the hippocampus, as well as maintenance of many neural functions across the nervous system. As discussed previously, imaging studies have described gray matter loss as a result of the excitotoxic effects of chronic stress as a radiological hallmark of burnout. Thus, it stands to reason that sBDNF levels may be influenced by burnout, and several studies have reported that sBDNF levels are significantly reduced in participants with burnout when compared with a control cohort without burnout.[18,19] In addition, there has also been more recent evidence to support an epigenetic role in the downregulation of BDNF production during burnout.[20] Although the apparent link between sBDNF expression and burnout is promising at this time, it is important to note that sBDNF levels modulate in a similar manner with other psychological conditions, such as major depressive disorder and posttraumatic stress disorder, once again highlighting the importance of a skilled clinical evaluation to properly interpret the results of testing biomarkers, such as these within the context of burnout.

Key Takeaways Regarding Neurobiology and Burnout

Burnout is a complex state of performance, and it can often be difficult to accurately identify. There is a nascent body of research investigating potential biomarkers for burnout; although some promising work has been presented, there are clear gaps that must be addressed before biomarkers alone can be confidently used. Burnout affects multiple bodily systems with overlap in clinical presentations, including posttraumatic stress disorder, depression, and anxiety. Thus, although these biomarkers may be useful, at this time, burnout is a clinical diagnosis, which is made even more challenging by the cyclical nature of the process. For a condition as multifactorial and complex as burnout, longitudinal studies with detailed multivariate analyses will be necessary.

MEASURING BURNOUT

The MBI was created to assess the 3 different theoretic components of burnout: emotional exhaustion, depersonalization, and reduced personal accomplishment. This instrument consists of 22 items that require participants to answer in terms of frequency (from 0, which is "never," to 7, which is "every day"). The MBI is not a direct measure of burnout, but a measure of the symptom constellation that makes up burnout. Subsequent tools were developed with varying degrees of acceptance, including the Eades Athlete Burnout Inventory (EABI).[21] However, the EABI contained conceptual and measurement limitations and has received criticism regarding its validity and reliability.[22]

Based on the authors' review of the literature, they recommend the Athlete Burnout Questionnaire (ABQ) which is a 15-item measure. The ABQ uses a 5-point Likert Scale comprising questions measuring the 3 subscales of athlete burnout (ie, physical and emotional exhaustion, sport devaluation, and reduced sense of accomplishment). **Table 1** provides examples of items included in the ABQ. Higher scores on the ABQ indicate more burnout. Research suggests this is both a reliable and a valid measure of athlete burnout.[22] Criticisms of the ABQ include concern that it is not a diagnosable measure of burnout and it does not obtain a dependable cutoff or way to classify burnout severity.

In the clinical evaluation, burnout must be distinguished from other behavioral, cognitive, and physical disorders. Cresswell and Eklund[3] reported that 2 separate measures used to measure athlete burnout, the ABQ and the MBI-GS can distinguish burnout from depression in athlete populations. However, this finding is far from conclusive, and clinicians must remember that conditions such as depression and burnout can coexist.

In summary, it is possible to assess for burnout; however, current assessment measures fall short on determining a clear threshold for the presence of burnout. The lack of a clear threshold is problematic in terms of accurate diagnosing, although more importantly, is less helpful in terms of treatment and prevention options. It is not clear when someone is experiencing burnout and/or at what level of severity.

Table 1
Example items on the Athlete Burnout Questionnaire and the associated symptoms

Symptom	Example Item	Almost Never		Sometimes		Almost Always
Sport devaluation	"I don't care about my sport performance as much as I used to"	1		2	3	4	5
Physical & emotional exhaustion	"I am exhausted by the physical and mental demands of sport"	1		2	3	4	5
Reduced sense of accomplishment	"I am not achieving much in sport"	1		2	3	4	5

Data from Raedeke TD, Smith AL. Development and preliminary validation of an athlete burnout measure. J Sport Exerc Psychol 2001; 23: 281-306.

Despite the current limitations of precise measurement of burnout, an approach using objective measures is recommended.

THE IMPACT OF BURNOUT ON ATHLETES

Burnout subscales created by Raedeke[8] provide an understanding of the short-term consequences of athlete burnout, but there is limited research on the long-term consequences. Short-term consequences include physical and emotional exhaustion, and these may carry into other areas of an athlete's life, including academics and social wellness. Physical exhaustion impedes training and performance; contributes to injury; and makes fully engaging in life outside of sports difficult. Emotional exhaustion can have a negative impact on motivation in sports and beyond.

Sport devaluation can also point to short-term consequences of athlete burnout. For many athletes, sports have served as a social engagement, which provides an opportunity for athletes to meet and connect with teammates, opponents, and others in the field of sports. Sports may also function as a coping strategy to deal with life stressors and adversity, as well as athletes' physical exercise that increases their physical well-being. A devaluation of performance could lead to sport discontinuation. The literature supports the idea that young athletes who experience burnout are less likely to participate as young adults because of early sport discontinuation.[23] Dropping out of sports could increase the risk of social isolation and decrease physical exercise. Athletes are also at risk of replacing their participation in sports, which served as a healthy outlet, with maladaptive behaviors. These losses may contribute to short-term negative consequences.

The last element of the 3 subscales and other short-term consequences to athlete burnout is a reduced sense of accomplishment. One of the many benefits of sports is that it provides athletes with a sense of accomplishment. Sports provide a setting in which athletes can monitor the growth of their skillset and experience mastery. Accomplishment can contribute to self-esteem and life satisfaction. A reduced sense of accomplishment may hinder these areas.

In addition to Raedeke subscales of athlete burnout, there are other consequences to burnout found in the literature. Burnout has been found to negatively impact sleep. It has been hypothesized that burnout is connected to the oversecretion of proinflammatory cytokines, which triggers the activation of the HPA axis, also known as the "stress system." The result of a stimulated HPA results in the secretion of epinephrine and norepinephrine. These 2 neurotransmitters play a role in the human body's fight-or-flight response to stress. Research has found burned-out individuals experience sleep disturbance consisting of difficulties falling asleep and not feeling refreshed after a night of sleep.[24]

MOTIVATION

The next step after developing a conceptual understanding of burnout as well as understanding how to identify and track it, is to understand the theoretic frameworks for prevention and intervention strategies. Motivation is a key component for both prevention and intervention of burnout; it can be thought of as a cognitive process that is pivotal to the burnout process. The cognitive process applied through Self-Determination Theory (SDT) is taking a wholistic approach instead of simply building skills. The goal of SDT is to increase motivation, while concurrently promoting psychological flourishing. SDT provides a helpful framework for prevention and intervention. As seen in **Fig. 2**, SDT focuses on the inner drive of motivation and presents (1) autonomy, (2) competence, and (3) relatedness as innate psychological needs. Autonomy provides athletes with choice, and this may have to be done in the context of a structured framework and/or demands; however, providing some opportunity for choice is powerful. Developing a sense of competence requires giving athletes challenges slightly beyond their current abilities. The challenges should not be too easy, leading to boredom, or too difficult, leading them to become overwhelmed. Finally, relatedness speaks to an athlete's need for connection and a sense of belonging, which is true for athletes that participate in team sports and individual sports. Athletes who develop a sense of connection with those around them learn to flourish in their environment.

Behaviors associated with autonomy, competence, and relatedness are found to act as protective factors from burnout for athletes and leads to psychological

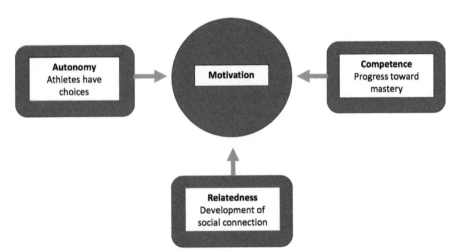

Fig. 2. The 3 pillars of the SDT. (*Data from* Deci EL, Ryan RM. The general causality orientations scale: Self-determination in personality. J Res Personality 2000;19: 109-134.)

flourishing. SDT distinguishes between different intrinsic (ie, participating in a behavior because of the personal fulfillment and joy it brings) and extrinsic motivation (ie, participating in a behavior because of the external factors, such as reward or recognition). Within the concept of extrinsic motivation, the SDT suggests varying degrees to the extent in which a behavior is autonomous. The goal for athletes is to maintain or increase intrinsic motivation, which can prevent burnout, whereas extrinsic motivation has a positive effect on burnout.

There is a link between athlete motivation and burnout. One study investigating elite athletes at the beginning and end of their seasons found that lower levels of self-determination at the beginning of a season was associated with higher levels of athlete burnout by the end of their season.[25] Conversely, athletes with higher levels of motivation were much less likely to report symptoms of burnout. Research has also found that motivation can fluctuate throughout the season, and athletes who experience a negative trend in their motivation throughout a season (ie, become less self-determined) were more vulnerable to developing symptoms on all 3 dimensions of burnout.

INTERVENTION AND PREVENTION

There are several factors that contribute to decreasing burnout and integrating them with concepts of motivation. When the links are clear, interventions can be created to promote psychological strength and concurrently reduce the risk of burnout.

Motivational Interventions

Motivation is the antithesis of burnout; thus, because of stark contrast between them, motivation can act as both a protective factor and a recovery method. Considering this relationship, providers can use interventions specifically geared toward enhancing athlete motivation levels. More specifically, interventions contribute to the enhancement of athlete's intrinsic motivation, including self-talk, mental imagery, and goal setting.

Self-Talk

Motivational self-talk enhances performance and assists athletes with perseverance in the face of performance obstacles (eg, fatigue, stress, muscles cramps).[26] Motivational self-talk is one's inner dialogue that contributes to increasing efforts, pushing through adversity, and ultimately enhancing overall motivation. It contributes to a sense of autonomy and sense of control; motivational self-talk is a reminder of what one is capable of. Although helpful in many different domains, motivational self-talk is most impactful during gross motor tasks (ie, endurance, strength). Regarding motivation, motivational self-talk has a positive influence on motivational-related outcomes, including self-confidence, effort, and cognitive anxiety. For this reason, athletes would benefit from developing awareness of their own personal self-talk as well as learning ways to implement motivational self-talk. It can also be used in a way that the athlete increases their focus on building competence rather than the outcome.

Mental Imagery

Mental imagery consists of the process of using the 5 senses (ie, vision, auditory, smell, touch, and taste) to consciously mimic a sensory skill. Engaging in mental imagery training increases the motivation of athletes to adhere to training programs, spend more time practicing, and maintain persistence. Athletes benefit from learning how to incorporate their senses into imagery to enhance vividness, and how to implement imagery into training. Learning a new way to enhance performance skills, envision ideal performance, and mentally prepare for potential performance adversity contributes to cultivating competence, although controlling performance within imagery and deciding which skills and elements of performance they are mentally rehearsing fosters autonomy.

Goal Setting

Goal setting is another technique that may benefit athletes from developing burnout and assist them in recovering from burnout. Setting goals provides athletes with something to work toward. Goals give athletes a sense of purpose each day in practice, allow them the opportunity to be intentional within their training, and require athletes to self-reflect, noticing their growth, their current skill set, and where they plan to go next. Goal setting not only increases intrinsic motivation but also contributes to other positive effects, including improvements in performance and increased effort.

Process goals are controllable milestones leading an athlete to their long-term goals (eg, stretch each night, focus on shooting form during free throw drill, get 8 hours of sleep each night). When athletes are focused on the process of their development as a result of setting process goals, they are more focused on the necessary step to achieve their goals, moving them toward competence. Providers can have a positive impact on athletes by assisting them in developing short- and long-term goals, as well as practice and competition goals that are both challenging and realistic. To enhance autonomy and motivation, providers should identify goals that athletes want to achieve for intrinsically motivated reasons rather than having goals that others (ie, coach, parents, teammates) have imposed.

Other Individual Interventions

There are additional individual interventions most likely linked to increasing motivation and ameliorating burnout, although there is no clear connection established in the literature.

Perfectionism

Perfectionism, a trait in which an individual does not accept any standard that is less than flawless, may create susceptibility to athlete burnout. Athletes with lower levels of perfectionism experience less exhaustion from sports participation (one of the consequences of burnout) in comparison to their more perfectionistic athlete peers.[27] Athletes who possess perfectionistic predispositions tend to have rigid perspectives associated with black or white thinking (eg, I either win this game or I am a failure). This type of thinking style makes it difficult for athletes to witness their own growth and successes outside of performance outcome. This form of rigidity can have a negative impact on experiencing joy from sport participation, harm confidence, and produce a fear of failure. Intervention at this level consists of assisting athletes in developing awareness of their perfectionistic thinking style as well as teach them strategies to begin to challenge and replace those thoughts.

Coping with Adversity

An athlete's ability to cope with adversity has a negative correlation with burnout. There are many demands and stressors that are unique to the athlete experience; those athletes who are better able to handle those demands are much less likely to experience burnout. Athletes who may not be well equipped to handle those demands are more vulnerable to stress, anxiety, and burnout.

Gratitude

Gratitude has been associated with lower levels of stress and burnout.[28] Because of the positive impact of gratitude, it would be beneficial for a sport psychologist to monitor an athlete's gratitude and encourage athletes to nourish their daily life gratitude to prevent or lessen the development of burnout.

Mindfulness

Mindfulness meditation is an effective intervention in alleviating both stress and burnout. Educating athletes on the various benefits of mindfulness in addition to teaching them techniques to make mindfulness a daily practice in their life could contribute to cultivating a resiliency toward athlete burnout.

ORGANIZATION

Prevention and intervention techniques targeting the individual athlete, although effective, are not sufficient to fully protect the athlete from burnout. Other techniques and considerations sport organizations and stakeholders may use to better support athletes are mentioned in later discussion.

Organizational Motivation Interventions and Prevention

There are specific things coaches and organizations can do to develop a motivational climate. For athletes, a motivational climate is the psychological environment in which they perform, prepare, and train. It is important to note that studies of motivational climate are based on athletes' perceptions, as opposed to the perspective of an objective outsider. Two motivational climates exist either separately or in combination: task-involving and ego-involving climates. As seen in **Table 2**, the task-involving climate emphasizes self-improvement, learning, growth, collaboration, and individual effort. On the other hand, an ego-involving climate occurs when athletes perceive an emphasis on success, outcomes, social comparison, and punishment for mistakes. Although elements of an ego-involving climate are important in specific circumstances, implementing a balance of task and ego with more emphasis on a task orientation can contribute to a more motivational climate. **Box 1** presents factors that create a motivational climate for athletes.

Table 2 Distinguishing the difference between a task-involving climate versus an ego-involving climate	
Task-Involving Motivation	**Ego-Involving Motivation**
Encourages self-improvement	Encourages being the best
Supports all athletes	Supports star athletes
Mistakes help athletes learn	Mistakes are not acceptable
Compete and learn from peers	Compare and compete with peers
Rewards effort	Rewards success

Data from Nordin-Bates SM, Raedeke TD, Madigan DJ. Perfectionism, burnout, and motivation in dance: A replication and test of the 2×2 model of perfectionism. J Dance Med Sci 2017; 21: 115-122.

Box 1
Factors that create a motivational climate for athletes

1. An environment in which athletes have some say in their training

2. Quality coaching relationships in terms of closeness, commitment, and complementarity

3. Autonomy supportive change-oriented feedback (ie, consists of an empathetic approach to providing descriptive feedback on behaviors that need modification for desired performance and problem-solving participation from the athlete)

4. Autonomy supportive promotion-oriented feedback (ie, consists of acknowledging and promoting observed desirable behavior/performances)

5. A shared belief in the team's ability to executive actions to produce a desired performance

---

SUMMARY

There is no diagnostic severity index or threshold that helps to identify an athlete as "burnt out." Similarly, neurophysiological biomarkers of burnout currently lack diagnostic sensitivity. Understanding the relationship between the 3 elements of motivation (autonomy, competence, and relatedness) and the 3 elements of burnout (sport devaluation, physical and emotional exhaustion, and reduced sense of accomplishment) is a key component to an athlete's performance success. The conceptualization of burnout in the context of sports is improving, as are the measures to assess for the presence of burnout. Motivation and the self-determination theoretic model serve as preventative and intervention measures for burnout. Future research needs to focus on the distinction between burnout and other mental health conditions; it needs to also investigate the diagnostic and management tools for addressing burnout and maximizing the athlete's performance.

Finally, the relationship between empathy and burnout is still largely undetermined. The use of empathy is not emphasized within the context of measuring athlete burnout; however, health care research reports that cultivating empathy can prevent burnout. The authors think that these incongruous findings are related to the fact that the value of empathy in preventing burnout is context dependent. Empathy directly impacts an athlete's ability to understand the experiences of others and to connect to teammates, coaches, and peers. However, in certain team cultures, this may not necessarily be advantageous, leading to an increased propensity for burnout. It is hoped that future research will elucidate the many factors related to burnout and help guide strategies for prevention, diagnosis, and treatment.

REFERENCES

1. National Collegiate Athletic Association. NCAA GOALS study of the student-athlete experience: initial summary of findings. 2016. Available at: http://www.ncaa.org/sites/default/files/GOALS_convention_slidebank_jan2016_p ublic.pdf. Accessed August 20, 2020.

2. Gustafsson H, Kenttä G, Hassmén P, et al. Prevalence of burnout in competitive adolescent athletes. Sport Psychol 2007;21:21–37.

3. Cresswell Scott L, Eklund RC. Athlete burnout: a longitudinal qualitative study. Sport Psychol 2007;21:1–20.

4. Maslach C, Jackson SE. The measurement of experienced burnout. J Organisational Behav 1981;2:99–113.

5. Smith RE. Toward a cognitive-affective model of athletic burnout. J Sport Psychol 1986;8:36–50.
6. Silva JM III. An analysis of the training stress syndrome in competitive athletics. J Appl Sport Psychol 1990;2:5–20.
7. Coakley J. Burnout among adolescent athletes: a personal failure or social problem? Soc Sci J 1992;9:271–85.
8. Raedeke TD. Is athlete burnout more than just stress? A sport commitment perspective. J Sport Exerc Psychol 1997;19:396–417.
9. Golonka K, Gawlowska M, Mojsa-Kaja J, et al. Psychophysiological characteristics of burnout syndrome: resting-state EEG analysis. Biomed Res Int 2019;2019: 3764354.
10. Luijtelaar G, vanVerbraak, Bunt M, et al. EEG findings in burnout patients. J Neuropsych Clin Neurosci 2010;22:208–17.
11. Tement S, Pahor A, Jaušovec N. EEG alpha frequency correlates of burnout and depression: the role of gender. Biol Psychol 2016;114:1–12.
12. Tei S, Becker C, Kawada R, et al. Can we predict burnout severity from empathy-related brain activity? Transl Psychiatry 2014;4:393.
13. Durning SJ, Costanzo M, Artino AR, et al. Functional neuroimaging correlates of burnout among internal medicine residents and faculty members. Fron Psych 2013;4:131.
14. Jovanovi H, Perski A, Berglund H, et al. Chronic stress is linked to 5-HT1A receptor changes and functional disintegration of the limbic networks. NeuroImage 2011;55:1178–88.
15. Golkar A, Johansson E, Kasahara M, et al. The influence of work-related chronic stress on the regulation of emotion and on functional connectivity in the brain. PLoS One 2014;9(9). https://doi.org/10.1371/journal.pone.0104550.
16. Savic I. Structural changes of the brain in relation to occupational stress. Cereb Cortex 2015;25:1554–64.
17. Chow YK, Masiak J, Mikołajewska E, et al. Limbic brain structures and burnout—a systematic review. Adv Med Sci 2018;63:192–8.
18. He S, Wu S, Wang C, et al. Interaction between job stress, serum BDNF level and the BDNF rs2049046 polymorphism in job burnout. J Affect Dis 2020;266:671–7.
19. Onen Sertoz O, Tolga Binbay I, Koylu E, et al. The role of BDNF and HPA axis in the neurobiology of burnout syndrome. Prog Neuro-Psychopharm Bio Psych 2008;32:1459–65.
20. Bakusic J, Ghosh M, Polli A, et al. Epigenetic perspective on the role of brain-derived neurotrophic factor in burnout. Trans Psych 2020. https://doi.org/10.1038/s41398-020-01037-4.
21. Eades AM. An investigation of burnout of intercollegiate athletes: the development of the Eades Athlete Burnout Inventory. Berkeley: University of California; 1990.
22. Raedeke TD, Smith AL. Development and preliminary validation of an athlete burnout measure. J Sport Exerc Psychol 2001;23:281–306.
23. Russell WD. The relationship between youth sport specialization, reasons for participation, and youth sport participation motivations: a retrospective study. J Sport Behav 2014;37:286.
24. Söderström M, Ekstedt M, Åkerstedt T, et al. Sleep and sleepiness in young individuals with high burnout scores. Sleep 2004;27:1369–77.
25. Lemyre PN, Treasure DC, Roberts GC. Influence of variability in motivation and affect on elite athlete burnout susceptibility. J Sport Exerc Psychol 2006;28: 32–48.

26. McCormick A, Meijen C, Marcora S. Effects of a motivational self-talk intervention for endurance athletes completing an ultramarathon. Sport Psychol 2018;32: 42–50.

27. Nordin-Bates SM, Raedeke TD, Madigan DJ. Perfectionism, burnout, and motivation in dance: a replication and test of the 2×2 model of perfectionism. J Dance Med Sci 2017;21:115–22.

28. Gabana NT, Steinfeldt JA, Wong YJ, et al. Gratitude, burnout, and sport satisfaction among college student-athletes: the mediating role of perceived social support. J Clin Sport Psychol 2017;11:14–33.

Anxiety
Recognition and Treatment Options

Vuong Vu, MD*, David Conant-Norville, MD

KEYWORDS

- Performance • Anxiety • Athletes • Sport Psychiatry • Mental health • Exercise
- Physical activity • Stress

KEY POINTS

- To recognize the unique stressors that athletes may face and how those may contribute to anxiety symptoms in their respective sport.
- To explore how anxiety symptoms can affect performance in sport.
- To identify appropriate non-pharmacologic and pharmacologic treatment strategies to assist athletes struggling with anxiety symptoms.

INTRODUCTION

According to the DSM-5, anxiety is the anticipation of future threats that are "excessive or persisting beyond developmentally appropriate periods" and "often associated with muscle tension and vigilance in preparation for future danger and cautious or avoidant behaviors."[1] The uneasiness experienced can generate a feeling of insecurity with an increase in physiologic activation, especially in the context of sports competitions.[2] Anxiety has also been shown to regulate the operation of attentional networks and may result in compromise of executive functioning and concentration, both of which may be influenced by "contextual sensitivity and vigilance processes."[3] With all of the aforementioned elements in mind, it can be postulated how anxiety symptoms can have a major effect on an athlete's performance.

Athletes experience anxiety symptoms at broadly similar rates to the general population but are faced with several unique factors that differentiate their experience.[2] Some mediators to consider that may affect anxiety across all ages and not unique to athletes include "childhood adversity, mastery, behavioral inhibition, ruminative style, neuroticism, physical health, physical activity, and perceived interpersonal and employment problems."[4] There also exist athlete-specific factors that may precipitate or exacerbate existing anxiety disorders including "pressure to perform and public scrutiny, career uncertainty or dissatisfaction, and injury."[2] Injury-associated

Mind Matters, PC, 10690 Northeast Cornell Road, Suite #315, Hillsboro, OR 97124, USA
* Corresponding author.
E-mail address: vvu@mindmatterspc.com

Psychiatr Clin N Am 44 (2021) 373–380
https://doi.org/10.1016/j.psc.2021.04.005
0193-953X/21/© 2021 Elsevier Inc. All rights reserved.

psych.theclinics.com

anxiety may be related to the injury itself or to the anxiety and concern of not being able to compete, which unfortunately can actually prolong the duration of recovery from injury.[5]

A 2018 meta-analysis found higher levels of competitive anxiety in female than in male athletes. The investigators cited a higher frequency of "oscillating levels of gonadal hormones" and the female tendency to more openly discuss their feelings/emotions as possible explanations.[6] The meta-analysis also found that younger athletes had "greater feelings of insecurity, emotional dependency and less use of elaborate coping strategies" when compared with older athletes, and athletes with greater experience have added ability to control their distress and have more "effective coping strategies to deal with criticism from oneself and others." In addition, an athlete's previous "poor performance tends to increase the levels of competitive anxiety" and is likely attributable to the "low level of self-confidence among athletes following a defeat."

A 2020 study further confirms findings that older age and experience on a national team (senior and youth levels) are associated with having less anxious characteristics and a more consistent stable response to stressful events.[7] "Somatic state anxiety" is the "physical/physiologic" expression of anxiety by athletes and is positively correlated with a fear of failure or internalizing worries. "Cognitive state anxiety" is the mental expression of anxiety by athletes and is negatively associated with hoping for success. An athlete's self-confidence level was negatively associated with having anxious personality traits.

Studies have also found there are higher levels of competitive anxiety for athletes partaking in individual sports compared with those on team sports.[6,8] When success depends solely on one person, as seen in individual sports athletes, there is increased anxiety in competition. With increased pressure to perform, there may be excessive focus on outcomes leading to more "internal attribution after failure" and further loneliness in doing so. The goal-oriented nature of many individual sports (eg, swimming, gymnastics, and running) may lead to hyperfocus on results (especially because success in these sports is often measured via a tallied number of points or a time), and participation in sports becomes more about producing results than actual enjoyment.

From a logistical standpoint, studies have also shown that "levels of competitive anxiety tend to increase before and during official competitions and in contests played away from home."[6] Away games are usually influenced by "travel, poor familiarity with [the other] venues, away supporters, referee bias and absence of family and social supports." A special consideration is in contests against opponents with close proximity (eg, nearby rivals) that may lead to increased anxiety, as there is often a hostile atmosphere with historical goals at stake in the matchup.

The 2018 meta-analysis cited earlier found no major difference in competitive anxiety levels between starting and reserve athletes; this finding is most likely because they are subject to the same level of training, routine, and results.[6] A smaller study of 128 athletes that focused on elite female football players did show that starting athletes had more robust self-confidence and thus less anxious features when compared with athletes who were seldom starters and with less playing time.[7] This study and the meta-analysis found no differences in the levels of competitive anxiety in different positions played or different sports—the studies specifically measured football, futsal, and basketball athletes.

When evaluating athletes for the potential presence of anxiety symptoms, a broad differential diagnosis must be considered because many conditions can present similarly and warrant varied treatment strategies (**Table 1**).

Table 1
Generalized anxiety disorder and its differential diagnosis

DSM-5 Criteria for GAD[1]:	Differential diagnosis to consider for anxiety symptoms in athletes (as distinctly separate conditions or comorbidities):

• Excessive anxiety and worry (apprehensive expectation), occurring more days than not for at least 6 mo, about several events or activities (such as work or school performance).
• The individual finds it difficult to control the worry.
• The anxiety and worry are associated with 3 (or more) of the following 6 symptoms (with at least some symptoms having been present for more days than not for the past 6 mo): Note: only one item is required in children.
  ○ Restlessness or feeling keyed up or on edge.
  ○ Being easily fatigued.
  ○ Difficulty concentrating or mind going blank.
  ○ Irritability.
  ○ Muscle tension.
  ○ Sleep disturbance (difficulty falling or staying asleep or restless, unsatisfying sleep).
	• Social anxiety disorder (including the performance specifier)
	• Panic disorder and panic attack specifier
	• Separation anxiety disorder
	• Obsessive compulsive disorder (OCD)
	• Obsessive-compulsive personality disorder (OCPD)
	• Specific phobias (eg, agoraphobia)
	• Posttraumatic stress disorder (PTSD)
	• Adjustment disorder with anxious mood
	• Substance- or medication-induced anxiety disorder
	• Anxiety disorder due to another medical condition
	• Attention-deficit hyperactivity disorder (ADHD)
	• Body dysmorphic disorder

DISCUSSION

Nonpharmacologic (eg, yoga, meditation, and exercise) and pharmacologic treatment protocols both play an important role in the management of anxiety, and recommendations vary based on the specific presentation and the severity of symptoms. Athletes presenting with mild to moderate anxiety symptoms often benefit from nonpharmacologic approaches, especially for those who prefer to not take medications. Pharmacologic choices are added in combination with nonpharmacologic strategies for athletes suffering from moderate to severe mental health symptoms but do come with side-effect profiles that may negatively affect athletic performance including, but not limited to, sleep disruption (eg, sedation or insomnia); weight gain or weight loss; cardiac side effects (including orthostatic hypotension, hypertension, tachycardia, palpitations, and arrhythmias); tremor or other motor changes (eg, akathisia or bradykinesia); impaired concentration; blurred vision or dizziness; and increased agitation.[9]

Nonpharmacological Recommendations

A multidisciplinary support team that includes a mental health provider is critical to maintaining peak performance in elite athletes.[10] In being part of the support network, the mental health provider often can assist the athlete in honing psychological attributes that are key to sustaining a high level of play such as "self-regulation, intrinsic motivation, self-confidence, effective coping skills, and a positive mindset." This support is particularly relevant to the younger and less experienced athlete who tends to struggle with greater competitive anxiety when compared with older and more experienced athletes, thus further supporting "the role of preventive or early intervention approaches in the management of anxiety disorders in athletes."[2]

When examining injury recovery in athletes, the other major psychological characteristic to consider is the concept of resilience and how it can encourage more constructive adjustments in harsh conditions. A review by Zurita-Ortega et al concluded that developing programs directed at improving resilience capacity can help "reduce anxiety during periods of injury, improve ability to prepare for stressful situations, reduce the recovery period and the likelihood of relapses in addition to increasing motivation during challenging events."[5]

Assisting athletes in developing positive adaptive strategies will assuredly aid them in managing their anxiety. Furthermore, early access and "youth-specific models of mental healthcare has resulted in decreased stigma and service barriers, improving access to evidence-based interventions" (eg, cognitive behavioral therapy [CBT]).[2] Athletes are especially well suited for psychotherapeutic interventions, given they usually show great discipline and are generally complicit with recommendations.[9] Effectiveness of different therapeutic modalities varies based on the athlete's symptom presentation and personality structure. Some examples include "graded exposure and behavioral experimentation [e.g., using thought records] for cases of social anxiety, response prevention for cases of OCD, and arousal reduction for those with GAD or panic disorder."[9] Readily available resources and support services for athletes transitioning out of sports (eg, retirement or injury) are important to have in place, given the possible risk factor of worsening anxiety from the presence and impact of recent adverse life events.[2]

Participation in organized sports has been found to be associated with "decreased risk of anxiety, increased self-esteem, and improved social abilities."[8] The social benefits of participating in sports have been linked to reduced stress and better self-reported overall mental health in young adults. In a more general sense, physical activity has been shown to be "inversely correlated with the incidence of anxiety disorders" and could be protective against anxiety disorders.[11] Meta-analyses have found that "exercise-based interventions can have a small or moderate effect on reducing the anxiety symptoms in people with anxiety disorders, [and this] anxiolytic benefit has also been found in people without a diagnosed anxiety disorder."[11] High levels of physical activity can be protective against depressive symptoms as well, which commonly co-occurs with anxiety disorders.[11]

Exercise may also diminish the stress response in a dose-dependent manner; "acute bouts of aerobic exercise prior to a psychosocial stress task significantly reduced systolic and diastolic blood pressure."[11] A recent small study looking at bowlers who actively increased their heart rate before throwing the bowling ball showed better bowling scores (compared with bowlers at rest before the throw), suggesting that the achieved reduction and overall greater change in heart rate contributed to lower chances of choking.[12] One study showed exercise training programs led to "reduced stress reactivity in cortisol levels, heart rate, and heart rate variability compared to a relaxation program."[11] In a different smaller study, acute exercise (as compared with subjects at quiet rest) reduced the state of feeling anxious after "exposure to arousing emotional stimuli," suggesting that acute exercise may protect one from the summative effects of anxious response to such stressors.[13]

Although there are less clear definitive results, yoga and other mindfulness-based interventions (eg, tai chi and qi gong) have shown evidence of positive effects for decreasing anxiety symptoms, particularly when used as adjunctive therapies.[14]

Pharmacologic Recommendations

Athletes suffering from moderate to severe anxiety symptoms may benefit most from a combination of nonpharmacologic and pharmacologic interventions. The side-effect profile and potential negative impact on the athlete's performance are among the chief considerations when selecting from the available anxiolytic medication options.

Although the selective serotonin reuptake inhibitors (SSRIs) have not directly been studied in the athlete population, a survey of Sport Psychiatrists reported a preference for using escitalopram, sertraline, and fluoxetine as first-line medications for treating a generalized anxiety disorder.[15] Buspirone was preferred behind the SSRIs by the Sport Psychiatrists, most likely due to a small study that demonstrated performance impairment via greater perceived exertion among recreational athletes, although notably only a single 45 mg dose was tested.[15,16] Nonetheless, buspirone is considered a generally safe medication that is not associated with dependence or addiction risks and is often used as an augmenting agent to help treat anxiety symptoms.[17]

Benzodiazepines can be useful in treating short-term severe anxiety and panic symptoms, but they are not the medications of choice for sport-related anxiety.[17] Benzodiazepines come with numerous side effects that are potentially detrimental to the athlete's health and performance that include, but are not limited to, sedation, cognitive blunting, dizziness, bradycardia, memory impairment, constipation, hypotension, and fatigue. In addition, they can lead to addiction and dependence.

The β-blockers (eg, propranolol) have been used in nonsport settings for performance anxiety (eg, musical performances or public speaking) but should be avoided in sports, as they may lower blood pressure in athletes who already may have relatively low blood pressures.[9,17,18] β-blockers may also inhibit performance in endurance athletes in decreased exercise tolerance via a lower cardiopulmonary capacity.[9,18] Given that β-blockers are effective in decreasing tremor and improving fine motor control, they may be perceived as performance-enhancing drugs and thus prohibited by the World Anti-Doping Agency in particular sports. β-blockers are prohibited at all times for athletes in archery and shooting but only prohibited in competition for billiards, automobile, darts, golf, and some events of skiing/snowboarding as well as underwater sports.[19]

Case Study

MK was a 15-year-old female springboard diver when referred to a Sport Psychiatrist because anxiety was impairing her ability to compete at a national and international level. She wanted to continue to compete in diving, and she had medaled in her first international competition in the prior year. Her success led to much more attention from the national diving organization and an opportunity to train with the national team. Shortly after her international success, she injured her right knee during practice. Subsequently, she could not return to her previous form. She was tentative coming off the board and could not get the spring she needed to finish her dives. Her new national coach told her she was not working hard enough and pushed her to "just work harder." An orthopedic consultation cleared her to return to training with a recommendation for physical therapy to strengthen her leg muscles.

She became preoccupied with fear of failure, constantly worried about her future in diving, and the opinions of her fellow national team divers. She felt anxious whenever she thought about training or competing. MK began to avoid training sessions. In school, because of her worry about diving, her ability to concentrate was impaired and school performance suffered. She reported that she felt she was "letting everybody down." She struggled to fall asleep at night due to ruminations about failing at diving. At the pool she often hyperventilated and felt lightheaded. When she would climb up to the 3-m springboard, she would often freeze and need to back down the ladder, which was embarrassing. Her confidence and competitive spirit left her. MK shifted her training to dryland only, eventually totally avoiding the pool.

MK had been an energetic and enthusiastic child. Growing up, her parents described her as cooperative and compliant. At age 8 years, she saw a competitive diving competition and declared that she wanted to be a diver. She learned quickly and displayed determination to continue until a new skill was mastered. Parents reported that her early coaches were warm, encouraging, and patient. MK became confident in diving and looked forward to local competitions. By age 12 years, she was winning regional age group competitions and had competed in national competitions. By age 14 years, she was invited to participate in the National Junior Olympic program and surprised all with top performances, leading to her opportunity to compete in an international competition.

MK's parents reported that her mental state had changed dramatically after her injury 8 months earlier. She had become apprehensive and avoidant not only during diving but in other realms of her life as well. MK described feeling restless and on edge. Her parents reported MK to be more irritable and frequently voicing multiple somatic complaints, specifically muscle tension, headache, tremor, and heart palpitation. They noted that her symptoms were impairing her social relationships, athletic performance, and academic functioning.

On the national team she had been assigned a coach who focused only on performance and who stressed perfection while often giving harsh criticism. MK had never experienced this type of "negative coaching." She revered her new coach for her past diving accomplishments and assumed her criticisms were proof that she (MK) could never compete at an international level again. She was afraid to talk to her coach about this fear. Her parents consulted the national diving organization administrator and were instructed to "let the coach coach."

After a thorough psychiatric assessment, MK was given the diagnosis of *Generalized Anxiety Disorder*. A treatment plan was developed to decrease MK's symptoms of anxiety, build her resilience, and learn new coping strategies. The first goal was to define symptoms of anxiety and teach relaxation techniques that she could practice at home. She was taught a 20-minute relaxation exercise and urged to practice it several times daily. This initial intervention helped MK to more quickly find a calmer state, but her confidence, poolside anxiety, school performance, and social relationships did not improve. MK entered weekly CBT, supplemented with a structured workbook and daily homework assignments. Efforts to consult with MK's coach about her condition and treatment were fruitless, as the coach was dismissive, stating, "everyone has anxiety." In consultation with the national diving organization administrator, MK was assigned a different coach.

Because MK's symptoms of anxiety were severe, she was started on fluoxetine, 20 mg. daily, and the dose was carefully increased to optimum benefit at 60 mg. daily, with no adverse effects. MK began to show improvement with decreased ruminations and decreased somatic symptoms. She learned to identify anxiety symptoms quickly and practice calming techniques. She started to actively challenge her anxious thoughts and reimagine her relationship with diving. MK returned to the pool and began to train regularly, under the guidance of her new coach who used a positive and encouraging coaching style. The first several coaching sessions focused on fundamentals of basic dives and then over the next 3 months more difficult dives were added.

MK regained her previous skills and a new growth mindset. She competed again at a regional and then at a national level, first as the junior, where she placed in the top 5. Her school performance recovered, and her social anxiety decreased in all settings.

Her coach noted her improved focus and dive execution during both training and competitions. At age 17 years, MK was invited to join the senior national team.

This case report highlights the complexity of managing an anxiety disorder in a developing elite athlete. A comprehensive assessment is important in order to understand the presenting symptoms in the context of the athlete's developmental history, temperamental characteristics, family psychiatric history, social and environmental influences, current stressors, physical injury and illness, and psychological and physical traumas. This case highlights the need to build a supportive and understanding team around the athlete, of family, friends, coaches, sports administrators, educators, medical personnel, and mental health specialists. Treating anxiety disorders in athletes requires building a predictable and evidence-based treatment plan. To build a trusting relationship, psychotherapy should be warm, supportive, and structured. For severe cases of anxiety, as this one, medication can play a necessary role in successful treatment.

SUMMARY

Athletes share similar stressors with the general population that may cause anxiety symptoms. However, mental health providers should consider athlete-specific factors as well such as injury, pressures to perform, and career dissatisfaction. The level of anxiety symptoms athletes may be facing can be influenced by several factors including an individual versus team sport, age, level of experience in their respective sport, and being a starter or reserve player. Anxiety can affect the athlete's sport performance and general livelihood. Mild to moderate anxiety symptoms should first be managed with nonpharmacologic strategies. Addition and combination with pharmacotherapy should be reserved for athletes struggling with moderate to severe anxiety symptoms.

CLINICS CARE POINTS

- A mental health provider can play a key role in assisting athletes combat anxiety symptoms via building up psychological characteristics such as self-confidence, effective coping skills, intrinsic motivation, and resilience.

- Different psychotherapy modalities (eg, cognitive behavioral therapy or exposure response therapy) can be helpful treating anxiety in athletes and may be supplemented with recreational levels of exercise, yoga, tai chi, and qi gong

- Although not directly studied in athletes, selective serotonin reuptake inhibitors are the first line choice of many Sport Psychiatrists when treating anxiety symptoms; buspirone may also be a good adjunctive medication to consider

- Most Sport Psychiatrists would not recommend using benzodiazepines to treat anxiety symptoms, given their negative side-effect profile.

- b-blockers should be used with caution in athletes, as they may lower blood pressure and cardiovascular efficiency and are prohibited by World Anti-Doping Agency in and/or out of competition for several sports.

DISCLOSURE

The authors have not declared a specific grant for this research from any funding agency in the public, commercial, or not-for-profit sectors. The authors have not declared any competing interests.

REFERENCES

1. APA - Diagnostic and Statistical Manual of Mental Disorders DSM-5 Fifth Edition. Available at: https://www.appi.org/Diagnostic_and_Statistical_Manual_of_Mental_Disorders_DSM-5_Fifth_Edition. Accessed October 19, 2020.
2. Rice SM, Gwyther K, Santesteban-Echarri O, et al. Determinants of anxiety in elite athletes: a systematic review and meta-analysis. Br J Sport Med 2019;53:722–30.
3. Pacheco-Unguetti AP, Acosta A, Callejas A, et al. Attention and anxiety: different attentional functioning under state and trait anxiety. Psychol Sci 2010;21(2): 298–304.
4. Leach LS, Christensen H, Mackinnon AJ, et al. Gender differences in depression and anxiety across the adult lifespan: The role of psychosocial mediators. Soc Psychiatry Psychiatr Epidemiol 2008;43:983–98.
5. Zurita-Ortega F, Chacón-Cuberos R, Cofre-Bolados C, et al. Relationship of resilience, anxiety and injuries in footballers: Structural equations analysis. PLoS One 2018;13(11):e0207860.
6. Rocha VVS, Osório FL. Associations between competitive anxiety, athlete characteristics and sport context: Evidence from a systematic review and meta-analysis. Rev Psiquiatr Clin 2018;45:67–74.
7. Madsen EE, Hansen T, Thomsen SD, et al. Can psychological characteristics, football experience, and player status predict state anxiety before important matches in Danish elite-level female football players? Scand J Med Sci Sports 2020;1–11.
8. Pluhar E, McCracken C, Griffith KL, et al. Team sport athletes may be less likely to suffer anxiety or depression than individual sport athletes. J Sport Sci Med 2019; 18:490–6.
9. Reardon CL, Hainline B, Miller Aron C, et al. Mental health in elite athletes: International Olympic Committee consensus statement (2019) Consensus statement. Br J Sport Med 2019;53:30.
10. Burns L, Weissensteiner JR, Cohen M. Lifestyles and mindsets of Olympic, Paralympic and world champions: is an integrated approach the key to elite performance? What are the findings? Br J Sport Med 2018;53:818–24.
11. Kandola A, Stubbs B. Exercise and anxiety. In: Advances in experimental medicine and biology, vol. 1228. Singapore: Springer; 2020. p. 345–52.
12. Hine K, Takano Y. Decreasing heart rate after physical activity reduces choking. Front Psychol 2020;11:550682.
13. Smith JC. Effects of emotional exposure on state anxiety after acute exercise. Med Sci Sports Exerc 2013;45(2):372–8.
14. Atezaz Saeed S, Cunningham K, Bloch RM. Depression and anxiety disorders: benefits of exercise, Yoga, and Meditation. Am Fam Physician 2019;99(10): 620–7. Available at: www.aafp.org/afp. Accessed November 9, 2020.
15. Reardon CL, Creado S. Psychiatric medication preferences of sports psychiatrists. Phys Sports Med 2016;44(4):397–402.
16. Marvin G, Sharma A, Aston W, et al. The effects of buspirone on perceived exertion and time to fatigue in man. Exp Physiol 1997;82(6):1057–60.
17. Patel DR, Omar H, Terry M. Sport-related performance anxiety in young female athletes. J Pediatr Adolesc Gynecol 2010;23(6):325–35.
18. Reardon CL. The sports psychiatrist and psychiatric medication. Int Rev Psychiatry 2016;28(6):606–13.
19. International Standard Prohibited List 2021. Available at: www.wada-ama.org. Accessed November 16, 2020.

Depression Assessment

Challenges and Treatment Strategies in the Athlete

Carla D. Edwards, MSc, MD, FRCP(C)

KEYWORDS

- Athlete • Sport • Psychiatry • Mental health • Depression • Mood

KEY POINTS

- Athletes can experience depression at similar rates as the general population; however, certain populations of athletes may develop depression at higher rates.
- Numerous sport- and nonsport-related risk factors can increase the likelihood of depression in athletes.
- There are numerous internal and external obstacles that can delay or prevent an athlete from seeking support for mental illness.
- Treatment strategies should have a functional focus and be shaped by a biopsychosocial formulation to incorporate the multidimensional aspects of depression in the athlete population.
- Psychotherapy is a first-line treatment of mild-to-moderate depression, but pharmacotherapy may be necessary for more severe illness.
- Sport- and athlete-specific considerations should inform choice of therapeutic agents to minimize negative impacts of pharmacotherapy.

INTRODUCTION

"Depression" can be a symptom of a state of being, a description of a mood, or a manifestation of a clinical disorder. Major depressive disorder (MDD) is an illness defined by the presence of a cluster of symptoms that results in significant functional impairment and can be classified as mild, moderate, or severe depending on the extent of impairment. The DSM 5 diagnostic criteria for MDD are listed in **Box 1**.[1]

MDD and other related disturbances in mood account for the highest proportion of psychiatric illnesses in the general population and are a leading cause of disability around the world. More than 300 million people suffer from depression, contributing to the global burden of morbidity and morality in all ages.[2,3] In 2015 the World Health Organization (WHO) estimated that nearly 6% of women and more than 4% of men

Department of Psychiatry and Behavioural Neuroscience, McMaster University, Hamilton, Ontario, Canada
E-mail address: Edwardcd@mcmaster.ca

Psychiatr Clin N Am 44 (2021) 381–392
https://doi.org/10.1016/j.psc.2021.04.011
0193-953X/21/© 2021 Elsevier Inc. All rights reserved.

psych.theclinics.com

Box 1
DSM 5 criteria for major depressive disorder (adapted from the DSM 5 Diagnostic and Statistical Manual of Psychiatric Disorders, American Psychological Association)

Major Depressive Disorder

A. Five (or more) of the following symptoms have been present during the same 2-week period and represent a change from previous functioning; at least one of the symptoms is either[1] depressed mood or[2] loss of interest or pleasure.

Note: do not include symptoms that are clearly attributable to another medical condition.

1. Depressed most of the day, nearly every day as indicated by subjective report (eg, feels sad, empty, hopeless) or observation made by others (eg, seems tearful) (*Note:* in children and adolescents, can be irritable mood)
2. Markedly diminished interest or pleasure in all, or almost all, activities most of the day, nearly every day (as indicated by subjective account or observation)
3. Significant weight loss when not dieting or weight gain (eg, change of more than 5% of body weight in a month) or decrease or increase in appetite nearly every day (*Note:* in children, consider failure to make expected weight gain)
4. Insomnia or hypersomnia nearly every day
5. Psychomotor agitation or retardation nearly every day (observable by others, not merely subjective feelings of restlessness or being slowed down)
6. Fatigue or loss of energy nearly every day
7. Feelings of worthlessness or excessive or inappropriate guilt (which may be delusional) nearly every day (not merely self-reproach or guilt about being sick)
8. Diminished ability to think or concentrate, or indecisiveness, nearly every day (either by subjective account or as observed by others)
9. Recurrent thoughts of death (not just fear of dying), recurrent suicidal ideation without a specific plan, or a suicide attempt or a specific plan for committing suicide

B. The symptoms cause clinically significant distress or impairment in social, occupational, or other important areas of functioning.

C. The episode is not attributable to the physiologic effects of a substance or to another medical condition
   Note: criteria A–C represent a major depressive episode.
   Note: responses to a significant loss (eg, bereavement, financial ruin, losses from a natural disaster, a serious medial illness or disability) may include the feelings of intense sadness, rumination about the loss, insomnia, poor appetite, and weight loss noted in criterion A, which may resemble a depressive episode. Although such symptoms may be understandable or considered appropriate to the loss, the presence of a major depressive episode in addition to the normal response to a significant loss should also be carefully considered. This decision inevitably requires the exercise of clinical judgment based on the individual's history and the cultural norms for the expression of distress in the context of loss.

D. The occurrence of the major depressive episode is not better explained by schizoaffective disorder, schizophrenia, schizophreniform disorder, delusional disorder, or other specified and unspecified schizophrenia spectrum and other psychotic disorders.

E. There has never been a manic episode or a hypomanic episode. Note: this exclusion does not apply if all of the maniclike or hypomaniclike episodes are substance-induced or are attributable to the physiologic effects of another medical condition.

Data from GBD 2017 Disease and Injury Incidence and Prevalence Collaborators. (2018). Global, regional, and national incidence, prevalence, and years lived with disability for 354 diseases and injuries for 195 countries and territories, 1990–2017: a systematic analysis for the Global Burden of Disease Study 2017. The Lancet. DOI. Retrieved November 15, 2020 from https://www.who.int/news-room/fact-sheets/detail/depression.

between the ages of 20 and 24 years experienced depression globally, with prevalence rates climbing annually in subsequent age intervals until the sixth decade for women and seventh decade for men. Depression was also identified as the major contributor to suicide.[4]

There is a common misperception that athletes are somehow immune to the harshest aspects of life, including mental illness. This misperception is created and perpetuated by society's tendency to idolize athletes and place them on pedestals, whereas multimillion dollar contracts and sponsorship deals serve to elevate the status of the athletes above the general population. Empirical studies have demonstrated that athletes are as likely to experience depression as the general population.[5–8]

Prevalence rates of depression in college athletes range from 15.6% to 25.6%,[5,6] and reported rates in college and elite athletes are typically higher in female athletes (which is consistent with the general population). The prevalence rates for depression in one studied group of elite athletes were consistent with WHO estimates as previously reported.[9]

RISK FACTORS FOR DEPRESSION IN ATHLETES

Depression develops from a complex interplay of biological, psychological, and social factors that can be influenced by adverse life events (eg, pandemics, unemployment, financial strain, losses, and trauma). Risk factors for depression in competitive athletes include female biological gender, freshman status in college, and pain.[10] Additional features that are associated with depression in athletes are described below:

1. Harassment, abuse, and trauma

   Athletes are human beings. They bring their histories with them wherever they go, which may include nonsport-related intentional violence such as sexual, physical, or psychological abuse as well as neglect. Preexisting mental illness can relapse, if conditions allow, at any point in an athlete's life. Nonaccidental violence is also prevalent in the world of sports, as described in the consensus statement by the International Olympic Committee in 2016.[11] The personal costs of nonaccidental violence can exist for many years and exert a significant amount of damage.[12] Athletes have self-reported anxiety, depression, low self-esteem and poor body image after a history of psychological abuse.[13]

2. Adverse childhood experiences (ACEs)

   ACEs are defined as potentially traumatic events that occur during childhood (before the age of 17 years).[14] Many athletes were raised in environments that undermined their sense of safety, stability, and bonding. They grew up in households that exposed them to violence, parents with mental illness, suicide, substance abuse, or instability caused by parental separation or incarceration. ACEs can be linked to chronic health problems, mental illness and substance abuse and can negatively affect lifestyle, education, and opportunities. Some children are at greater risk than others, as women and several racial and ethnic minority groups are at greater risk for having experienced 4 or more types of ACEs. Often, sports create opportunities for athletes to "escape" adverse, violent, suppressive, or oppressive life situations. As they find success in the world of sports, they often carry the burden of responsibility to support their families who continue to live under those conditions.

3. Genetics

Athletes with a family history of mood disorder have an increased risk of developing a mood disorder. The lifetime prevalence of major depression in the general population is 10% to 15%; however, first-degree relatives have a 2- to 3-fold increase in risk of developing depression.[15]

4. Environmental factors

Athletes experience a multitude of unique environmental and lifestyle factors that may influence their mood state. Those who follow a high-performance pathway from their youth may leave their family homes at a young age and live far away from their families in pursuit of their dreams in the sport world. Some sports require their athletes to travel the world throughout the calendar year to accumulate points for World Cup or Olympic qualification, and some stay at their temporary "home base" for no longer than 2 weeks at any given time. Relationship challenges, time zone shifts, lack of consistent support base, and the stress of a nomadic lifestyle for numerous sports can take its toll over time.

5. Commodification

Commodification of athletes as assets as opposed to individuals with rights increases the risk of their personal needs and rights being neglected or invalidated.[11] Young athletes learn from an early age that they have higher value if they are healthy and "not damaged." They are "expendable" if injured, ill, or underperform. In professional sports (as well as their developmental pathways), athletes are traded, moved, and shuffled in accordance with the organization's needs. This can lead an athlete to question their value and importance. When this occurs with young athletes who have left home to enter high-performance developmental leagues during adolescence, one can hypothesize that there would be an impact on the formation of their identity, sense of self, maturity, and self-efficacy. Frequent relocations, lack of "job security," being pawns in the business side of sport, and chasing a dream that may never be within reach can be devastating and result in significant mood disturbance.

6. Failure-based and situational depression; postcompetition "crash"

Sports crown champions and brand losers.[16] Sports-related failures can be so profound that they lead to depression and suicide.[17] Failure in sports can take many forms, including not being selected to a team, losing a championship game, match, bout, or race, or not performing well "when they had their shot." When the athlete's whole identity is entrenched in their "athletic persona," lack of success can lead these athletes to feel hopeless, alone, and many feel like they cannot even go on living their lives. After losing to Holly Holm in an Ultimate Fighting Championship bout in 2016, mixed martial artist and previous champion Ronda Rousey stated "What am I anymore if I am not this?" She described sitting the corner of the medical room pondering suicide after losing the fight.[18]

The magnitude of the athlete's response to sport failure will be quite individualized, based on their personal histories, past successes, stage of career, past management of losses, and how tightly their identities are tied to their accomplishments. Some athletes fear the loss of identity, purpose, relevance, and value in the wake of a loss. Depression rates in elite athletes are higher in the aftermath of poor performance and a subsequent sport-failure experience.[19]

Although numerous stressors affect athletes, including performance execution, maintaining health and healthy lifestyles, balancing academics, rehabilitating injuries, facing retirement, adjusting to success, managing performance expectations, and anxiety; failure in competition is the one stressor that seems to increase negative affect and mood disorders such as depression.[19]

Athletes on high performance or elite trajectories dedicate the bulk of their adolescence and young adulthood training for World Championships and Olympic Games. The sacrifices made along the way include relationships, education, employment, friendships, and deferral of establishing new families. Often, relationships do not survive the intensity of training, frequency of travel, and extent of commitment to sports that is required of prospective Olympians or professional athletes.

To many, the Olympics Games is "the pinnacle" of their dreams and aspirations. Athlete experiences at the Olympics are extremely variable. Success can result in elation, euphoria, confidence, and opportunities for sponsorship and endorsements. Unfortunately, there are many more athletes who do not win medals or do not perform as hoped. Some miss the podium by 0.01sec, despite thousands of hours of training and countless miles traveled around the world during the quadrennial of preparation. Some athletes experience collisions, crashes, or injuries that derail their dreams.

However their Olympic experience plays out, the amount of *themselves* that the athletes contribute to their journey leaves an indelible mark that irreversibly affects their identity, sense of self, and purpose. Regardless of success or failure, many Olympians experience a "postgames crash" when the quadrennial comes to an end; and they are faced with significant decisions. These include starting again for the next quadrennial, taking a break and experiencing life as they consider their future options, or moving on with "regular" life beyond that of an elite athlete. In the 4- to 6-week period immediately following a Major Games, athletes can experience a drop in their mood, energy, and motivation and may question their future directions. It stands to reason that this is a time during which athletes would benefit from increased mental health supports.

7. The unanticipated burden of success

Athletes train for the better part of 4 years to compete for Olympic glory. They later focus on performance and outcomes with exposure to international competition along the way at World Championships, World Cups, Pan American Games, Commonwealth Games, and others. Although many athletes are long shots for medals, others are identified as favorites to win certain events.

Athletes train and compete with the goal of winning. Some athletes with unbridled potential surprise the world with unanticipated podium performances, sometimes coming at a very young age. At the 2016 Rio Olympic Games, 16-year-old Canadian swimming prodigy Penny Oleksiak shocked the swimming world by becoming Canada's youngest Olympic gold medalist, as well as the first Canadian athlete to win 4 Olympic medals at a single Olympic Games. She was selected to be the Flag Bearer at the Closing Ceremonies of the Games and later that year won the Lou Marsh Award as Canada's Athlete of the Year and the Bobbie Rosenfeld Award as the CP Female Athlete of the Year.

Imagine the changes in that athlete's life experience: sudden influx of sponsorship deals, requests for interviews, and public speaking opportunities. That athlete's experience of their status in national sports suddenly thrusts them at the forefront of all media highlights and stories, and their names are mentioned as favorites to win subsequent competitions.

Athletes train to win; but they are not often taught the skills to manage the challenges that accompany success. Sometimes athletes can internalize their successes to fuel self-belief and confidence as they proceed with their training, whereas others become paralyzed by their success and are intimidated by challengers even within their own program. Depression and anxiety can manifest in an athlete who feels that they cannot sustain their previous levels of success, particularly if the media sets the stage for that expectation. Athletes have described feeling the burden that they are carrying the country on their shoulders and are fearful that they will let "the country down" with sub-par performances. This self-doubt and prediction of negative appraisal set the stage for a spiral of self-doubt, decreased performance, increased self-comparison with others, and anticipation of the criticism they will receive in the media. These elements can weigh quite heavily on these athletes.

8. Injuries

Physical injuries can be devastating for athletes. Pivotal factors such as nature and severity of the injury, timing (relative to playoffs or major competition), impact on career, likelihood of returning to preinjury success, and duration of training interruption may have a significant impact on mental health.[16] Injuries can also place athletes at a higher risk of suicide. Characteristics that increase suicidal risk include preinjury success, requiring surgical intervention, lengthy recovery and rehabilitation process, prolonged sport interruption, inability to attain preinjury levels of success, and loss of position.[17,20]

Stress is an antecedent to injury and can influence an athlete's response to injury and their approach to rehabilitation and recovery.[21] Mental illness can be triggered or unmasked by maladaptive response to injury, including anxiety, depression, disordered eating, and substance use disorders. When access to sports is interrupted by injury, athletes may lose their outlet for stress as well as their means of expressing their talents, energy, and emotions.[16] When their overall identity is tied to their athletic performance, the injured athlete may struggle with their purpose and sense of being.[22]

9. Traumatic brain injury (TBI)

Concussion is the most common head injury in young adults and the most frequently type of head injury sustained in sports.[23,24] The Center for Disease Control and Prevention (CDC) in the United States estimated an annual occurrence of concussions between 1.6 and 3.8 million in sports and recreational activities[25]; however, the true incidence is likely much larger because as much as 50% of concussions go unreported.[26] The constellation of heterogeneous symptoms associated with concussions span physical (headache, dizziness, neck pain), cognitive (memory impairment, poor concentration and attention, executive function challenges, word finding difficulties, cognitive fatigue, difficulty with problem solving and multitasking), affective (depression, anxiety, emotional regulation, irritability, adjustment reaction), sensory (sensitivity), vestibular dysfunction, and oculomotor changes.[27]

TBIs have been linked with mental illnesses such as major depression, generalized anxiety disorder, suicide, and other chronic neuropsychiatric sequelae.[23,25] Although most of those who sustain concussions recover without lingering effects, 10% to 20% of concussion sufferers have persistent, prolonged, complicated, or incomplete recoveries.[28–30] Mental disorders may occur at higher rates in concussion sufferers. The development of mental health challenges, including depression and anxiety, following concussions may negatively affect recovery.[31,32]

Individuals who have sustained head injuries have a greater frequency of suicide attempts and a higher risk of death by suicide than those who have not experienced head injuries.[33] Suicidal behavior may increase if mental health symptoms are not addressed following a head injury.[27] In addition to mood, anxiety, and psychotic disorders that can result from head injuries, the impact of life changes that result from physical and neurocognitive impairment can be extremely challenging or even catastrophic. Sports are often a cathartic outlet for athletes and for many their athletic personas define them. Missing entire (or multiple) seasons or being medically advised to not return to their sport can result in a transitional crisis.

The association of concussion with mental illness and suicide should prompt regular screening of every athlete presenting with mental illness for a history of head trauma and vice versa.

10. Retirement

Retirement from high-performance sports represents a major life transition for many athletes who have dedicated most of their adolescence and young adulthood to training and competition. For many athletes who compete at the level of international games (including World Championships and Olympic/Paralympic Games), their sport is their job and training consumes more of their waking hours than would most professions. For professional athletes, their sport performance is their profession.

When an athlete's identity is fully entrenched in their athletic persona and image, any changes to that entity has the potential to cause concerning challenges to mental health and function.

Studies have demonstrated that the prevalence of anxiety and depression in athletes transitioning out of sport approaches 45%.[34–36] The context of this transition may have some influence on the emotional impact, as planned retirement "on the athlete's terms" may enable the athlete to establish a degree of preparedness versus those who are ushered from their sport before they are ready either by injury or "deselection."[37–39] Additional factors that may contribute to the development of mental health challenges in the context of transition out of sport include high levels of athletic identity, lower educational attainment, lack of retirement planning, adverse life events, chronic pain, and postretirement unemployment.[40–42]

Most athletes adjust to life beyond their competitive career within 2 years; however, even planned transitions out of sport can result in crisis for some.[43] The integrated support team (IST) that supports athletes during their careers can also assist in preparing them for the transition. This may include nutritionists, strength and conditioning coaches, physiologists, mental performance consultants, clinical psychologists, and Sport Psychiatrists. Intrinsic skills such as organization, finding purpose, accessing creativity, academic inquisitiveness, and forward thinking can also assist in the transition.

Protection and promotion of mental health in elite and professional athletes during their careers and before retirement may mitigate the impact of transition from sport. Initiatives such as Game Plan,[44] the National Football League (NFL) "Play Smart Play Safe" program,[45] and the National Basketball Players Association (NBPA) Player Wellness Program[46] have developed specific programming to help their athletes access education, financial strategies counseling, and retirement planning *before* they transition from sport. As such, these programs seek to mitigate the impact of retirement and equip the athletes with the foundational skills to find success beyond their sporting careers.

POTENTIAL OUTCOMES

It has already been stated that athletes are vulnerable to the same mental illnesses as the general population. It stands to reason that they would also be at risk for the same sequelae of depression as the general population. Mild depression can manifest as low mood, reduced drive and motivation, and low self-esteem. Advancing along the more severe end of the illness could introduce further impairments such as sleep disturbance, low energy, lack (or increase) of appetite, weight loss (or gain), hypersomnolence, social withdrawal, poor concentration, guilt, psychomotor retardation, and suicidal ideation.

Athletes with depression experience impairment both in their sports world and their "regular" life. Depression can affect psychological and physical health, relationships, and performance. Without timely and accurate assessment and treatment, depression manifestation could be misinterpreted as laziness, bad attitude, bad behavior, disengagement, lack of commitment, or lack of effort, which could result in athletes being inaccurately "labeled," losing sport opportunities, and being ostracized by their sport body.

Timely assessment would provide the athlete with appropriate investigation of potential medical causes of their symptoms, diagnosis, and multimodal management.

OBSTACLES TO ASSESSMENTS

Athletes are more likely to see a physician about physical symptoms or injury than symptoms of psychological distress. Building mental performance strategies are an accepted element of sports and is unlikely to have stigma attached. Accessing support for mental health is often challenging for athletes, and there are many reasons for this:

1. Lack of regular screening, resources for interpretation, and follow-up: screening for mental illness is not uniformly part of preparticipation questionnaires or examinations. Further, staff who are tasked with implementing preparticipation screening typically do not have the background skills or training to identify or respond to mental illness indicators.
2. Lack of qualified mental health personnel with sports organizations: most sport organizations do not have a comprehensive mental health and performance team. There is a relative abundance of mental performance personnel as compared with mental health clinicians (including psychologists and psychiatrists), as the sports world is still evolving to recognize that mental health is part of performance, and without mental health, peak performance is not attainable.
3. Stigma: athletes fear being labeled as "weak," "defective," or "unreliable" because of mental illness. Fear of lost opportunities due to unfair judgment also influences an athlete's openness to seek and receive support for mental illness. Although there has been an increasing trend of high-profile athletes publicly disclosing their struggles with mental illness, disclosure of mental illness may make some athletes vulnerable to bullying and harassment based on their illness. In addition, elite, high-performance and professional athletes often rely on sponsorship, marketing, and financial incentives to provide supplemental income for

their livelihood. They may fear loss of financial support that would accompany identification of mental illness.

4. Avoidance: elite and high-performance athletes are driven by goals, demanding training programs, travel, and competitions. There is rarely "down time." Attendance to mental health concerns may be assumed or perceived to be time-consuming and emotionally taxing (which may be interpreted as inconvenient and unnecessary as they pursue their goals). As such, psychological struggles may be "put aside," avoided, or ignored as long as possible.

5. Fear of sports-based repercussion or bias (particularly if there is a lack of return-to-play pathway for training interrupted by mental illness): similar to stigma, athletes fear loss of sport opportunities if they are labeled as having mental illness. Missed training or competitions due to mental illness may create discomfort and uncertainty within the sport organization regarding the athlete's ability to return to play. Without a comprehensive mental health and performance team to guide education of the IST and return to train parameters, athletes with mental illness may be unfairly excluded from training and competition.

6. Image: intentional or not, high-profile athletes have an image in society that is created by their appearance, performance, social behavior, lifestyle, and accomplishments. They may perceive that acknowledging the presence of mental illness would tarnish their image or result in them losing social commodity.

TREATMENT STRATEGIES

Assessment of mood symptoms in an athlete should include biopsychosocial formulation to enable the identification of the multifaceted elements that can contribute to mood changes in this population. This approach would allow the assessor to identify risk factors (predisposing) that were outlined earlier in this chapter, in addition to precipitating and perpetuating elements from multiple dimensions. Athletes are incredibly resilient individuals, and identification of their protective factors can assist in the development of multimodal treatment strategies that can engage the athlete as a partner.

Recognizing the athlete as an active individual with multiple high-pressure demands is important in approaching treatment with a functional focus. In contrast with the conventional approach to mental illness in the general population in which exposure to stressors is minimized, management of depression and other mental illnesses in athletes typically requires a parallel process with their continued involvement in sport (although this may require modification in the event of severe mental illness).

Treatment of depression in athletes may include psychotherapy with or without concurrent medication management. Psychotherapy, or "talk therapy," engages the athlete in exploration of psychological challenges using therapeutic principles, structure, and techniques.[47] Psychotherapy can be delivered by professionals such as social workers, psychotherapists, counselors, psychologists, and psychiatrists.

For individuals with more severe mental illness, pharmacotherapy may be indicated. Consideration of any medication use in an elite or professional athlete should be accompanied by reviewing potential agents with the World Anti-Doping Agency list of prohibited substances and methods.[48] Choice of pharmacologic agents for athletes should include careful consideration of side effects that could negatively affect athletic performance, including sedation, weight gain, weight loss, cardiac side effects, vision changes, or neurocognitive changes.[47] There is a paucity of randomized control trials (RCTs) of antidepressant medications with athletes, but the published RCTs demonstrated no adverse performance outcomes as a result of treatment with fluoxetine, paroxetine, or bupropion.[7] Surveys of prescribing preferences by Sport Psychiatrists indicated that most of them (63%) prescribed fluoxetine, followed by venlafaxine (21%).[49] Reasons cited for preference of fluoxetine included its activating properties and lack of influence on weight.

CLINICS CARE POINTS

- Exploration of social history in athletes should include areas that may reflect an increased risk for development of depression, including history of harassment, abuse and trauma, adverse childhood experiences, and environmental factors.

- Understanding an athlete's response to negative sport experiences or adjustment following major sporting events can enhance preparation and supports at key points in the athlete's career.

- Screening for depression should be implemented with the occurrence of injuries, retirement, or major life changes to facilitate early identification and management.

- Management approaches to treating depression in athletes should follow a biopsychosocial construct, with considerations for training, competition and antidoping regulations.

DISCLOSURE

The author has no financial or other conflicts of interest to declare.

REFERENCES

1. American Psychiatric Association. Diagnostic and statistical manual of mental disorders (DSM-5). Washington, DC: American Psychiatric Publishing; 2013.
2. GBD 2017 Disease and Injury Incidence and Prevalence Collaborators. Global, regional, and national incidence, prevalence, and years lived with disability for 354 diseases and injuries for 195 countries and territories, 1990–2017: a systematic analysis for the Global Burden of Disease Study 2017. Lancet 2018; 392(10159):1789–858. Available at: https://www.who.int/news-room/fact-sheets/detail/depression. Accessed November 15, 2020.
3. Liu Q, Hairong H, Yang J, et al. Changes in the global burden of depression from 1990-2017: findings from the global burden of disease study. J Psychiatr Res 2020;126:134–40.
4. Depression and other common mental disorders: global health estimates. Available at: http://apps.who.int/iris/bitstream/handle/10665/254610/WHO-MSD-MER-2017.2-eng.pdf. Accessed February 18, 2019.
5. Wolanin A, Hong E, Marks D, et al. Prevalence of clinically elevated depressive symptoms in college aged athlete and difference by gender and sport. Br J Sports Med 2016;50:167–71.
6. Wolanin A, Gross M, Hong E. Depression in athletes: prevalence and risk factors. Curr Sports Med Rep 2015;14(1):56–60.
7. Reardon C, Factor R. Sports psychiatry: a systematic review of diagnosis and medical treatment of mental illness in athletes. Sports Med 2010;40(11):961–80.
8. Rice SM, Purcell R, De Silva S, et al. The mental health of elite athletes: a narrative systematic review. Sports Med 2016;46:1333–53.
9. Gulliver A, Griffiths K, Mackinnon A, et al. The mental health of Australian elite athletes. J Sci Med Sport 2015;18:255–61.

10. Yang J, Peek-Asa C, Corlette JD, et al. Prevalence and risk factors associated with symptoms of depression in competitive collegiate student athletes. Clin J Sport Med 2007;17(6):481–7.

11. Mountjoy M, Brackenridge C, Arrington M, et al. International Olympic Committee consensus statement: harassment and abuse (non-accidental violence) in sport. Br J Sports Med 2016;50:1019–29.

12. Tofler I, Morse EE. Interface between sport psychiatry and sports medicine. Clin Sports Med 2005;24:4.

13. Stirling AE, Kerr GA. The perceived effects of elite athletes' experiences of emotional abuse in the coach-athlete relationship. Int J Sport Exerc Psychol 2013;11:87–100.

14. Available at: https://www.cdc.gov/violenceprevention/aces/fastfact.html?CDC_AA_refVal=https%3A%2F%2Fwww.cdc.gov%2Fviolenceprevention%2Facestudy%2Ffastfact.html. Accessed November 16, 2020.

15. Lohoff FW. Overview of the genetics of major depressive disorder. Curr Psychiatry Rep 2010;12(6):539–46.

16. Edwards CD, Berlin JS. The psychiatric emergency care of VIPs and athletes in crisis. In: Emergency psychiatry: principles and practice. Philadelphia: Wolters Kluwer; 2021. p. 459–69.

17. Baum AL. Suicide in athletes: a review and commentary. Clin Sports Med 2005; 24:853–69.

18. Griggs B. "Ronda Rousey: I thought about killing myself." *CNN.* 2016. Available at: https://www.cnn.com/2016/02/17/entertainment/ronda-rousey-feat/index.html. Accessed February 18, 2019.

19. Hammond T, Gialloreto C, et al. The prevalence of failure-based depression among elite athletes. Clin J Sport Med 2013;23(4):273–7.

20. Smith AM, Milliner EK. Injured athletes and the risk of suicide. J Athl Train 1994; 29(4):337–41.

21. Putukian M. The psychological response to injury in student athletes: A narrative review with a focus on mental health. Br J Sports Med 2016;50:145–8.

22. Masten R, Strazar K, Zilavec I, et al. Psychological response of the athletes to injury. Kinesiology 2014;46(1):127–34.

23. Fralick M, Thiruchelvam D, Tien HC, et al. Risk of suicide after concussion. CMAJ 2016;188(7):497–504.

24. Esfandiari A, Broshek D, Freeman JR, et al. Psychiatric and neuropsychological issues in sports medicine. Clin Sports Med 2011;30:611–27.

25. Finkbeiner NW, Max JE, Longman S, et al. Knowing what we don't know: long-term psychiatric outcomes following adult concussion in sports. Can J Psychiatry 2016;61(5):270–6.

26. Harmon KG, Drezner JA, Gammons M, et al. American Medical Society for Sports Medicine position statement: concussion in sport. Br J Sports Med 2013;47: 15–26.

27. Kontos AP, Deitrick JM, Reynolds E. Mental health implications following sport-related concussion. Br J Sports Med 2016;50(3):139–40.

28. Mooney G, Speed J. The Association Between Mild Traumatic Brain Injury and Psychiatric Conditions. Brain Inj 2001;15:865–77.

29. Epstein RS, Ursano RJ. Neuropsychiatry of traumatic brain injury. Washington, DC: American Psychiatric Press; 1994.

30. Solomon GS, Kuhn AW. Depression as a modifying factor in sport-related concussion: a critical review of the literature. Phys Sportsmed 2015;44:14–9.

31. Corwin DJ, Zonfrillo MR, Master CL, et al. Characteristics of prolonged concussion recovery in a pediatric subspecialty referral population. J Pediatr 2014; 165:1207–15.
32. Lange RT, Iverson GL, Rose A. Depression strongly influences postconcussion symptom reporting following mild traumatic brain injury. J Head Trauma Rehabil 2011;26:127–37.
33. Wasserman L, Shaw T, Vu M, et al. An Overview of Traumatic Brain Injury and Suicide. Brain Inj 2008;22(11):811–9.
34. Prinz B, Dvořák J, Junge A. Symptoms and risk factors of depression during and after the football career of elite female players. BMJ Open Sport Exerc Med 2016; 2:e000124.
35. Gouttebarge V, Kerkhoffs G, Lambert M. Prevalence and determinants of symptoms of common mental disorders in retired professional rugby union players. Eur J Sport Sci 2016;16:595–602.
36. Gouttebarge V, Aoki H, Kerkhoffs GM, et al. Prevalence and determinants of symptoms related to mental disorders in retired male professional footballers. J Sports Med Phys Fitness 2016;56:648–54.
37. Brown J, Kerkoffs G, Lambert MI, et al. Forced retirement from professional rugby union is associated with symptoms of distress. Int J Sports Med 2017;38:582–7.
38. Sanders G, Stevinson C. Associations between retirement reasons, chronic pain, athletic identity, and depressive symptoms among former professional footballers. Eur J Sport Sci 2017;17:1311–8.
39. Wippert P-M, Wippert J. The effects of involuntary athletic career termination on psychological distress. J Clin Sports Psychol 2018;4:133–49.
40. Knights S, Sherry E, Ruddock-Hudson M. Investigating elite end-of-athletic-career transition: a systematic review. J Appl Sport Psychol 2016;28:291–308.
41. Van Ramele S, Aoki H, Kerkhoffs G, et al. Mental health in retired professional football players: 12-month incidence, adverse life events, and support. Psychol Sport Exerc 2017;28:85–90.
42. Schuring N, Aoki H, Gray J, et al. Osteoarthritis is associated with symptoms of common mental disorders among former elite athletes. Knee Surg Sports Traumatol Arthrosc 2017;25:3179–85.
43. Available at: https://sirc.ca/blog/athlete-transition-out-of-sport/. Accessed November 22, 2020.
44. Available at: https://www.mygameplan.ca/about/mission-history. Accessed November 21, 2020.
45. Available at: https://www.playsmartplaysafe.com/resource/total-wellness/. Accessed November 21, 2020.
46. Available at: https://nbpa.com/offthecourt/transition-conversations. Accessed November 21, 2020.
47. Reardon CL, Hainline B, Miller Aron C, et al. Mental health in elite athletes: International Olympic Committee consensus statement (2019). Br J Sports Med 2019; 53:667–99.
48. Available at: https://www.wada-ama.org/en/content/what-is-prohibited. Accessed November 22, 2020.
49. Baum AL. Psychopharmacology in athletes. In: Sports psychiatry. New York (NY): WW Norton & Company, Inc.; 2000. p. 249–59.

Sleep Disorders in the Athlete

Shane A. Creado, MD[a,*], Shailesh Advani, MD, PhD[b]

KEYWORDS

• Athletes • Sport Psychiatry • Performance • Mental health • Sleep

KEY POINTS

• Athletes have unique characteristics and sleep needs compared with the general population, and therefore, specific sleep screening tools and strategies are indicated.
• There is a great need for a multidisciplinary collaborative approach to develop effective strategies to promote sleep health among athletes and sports professionals.
• Understanding the integrated roles or sleep, mental health, and sports performance will help to bridge the gaps in health care delivery to athletes.
• There remains a critical need to develop educational interventions to raise awareness among stakeholders in the sports world on the impact of sleep disturbances on mental health issues and sports performance.
• There needs to be a collective effort in the sports world to create sleep guidelines and resources for athletes, teams, and sports organizations.

INTRODUCTION

The prevalence of sleep disorders continues to increase in the United States and tends to have a detrimental impact on the overall health and quality of life in the general population. These sleep disorders include insomnia, sleep apnea, circadian rhythm disorders, hypersomnias, and parasomnias. Other factors that may contribute to sleep disorders include digestive issues, pain, medications, and mental health problems. An estimated 4% to 22% of adults in the United States meet diagnostic criteria for insomnia.[1] Furthermore, sleep apnea remains a common condition that affects at least 10% of the adult US population. In parallel to the general population, sleep disorders are a significant concern for many top athletes.

As the field of Sport Psychiatry evolves, awareness of sleep disorders among athletes is increasing as well as the importance of proactively addressing its impact on performance. Evidence suggests that athletes experience inadequate sleep at higher rates as compared with the general population: For example, compared with

[a] 625 West Madison Street, Apartment 4111, Chicago, IL 60661, USA; [b] National Institutes of Health
* Corresponding author.
E-mail addresses: shanecreado@gmail.com; info@shanecreado.com

Psychiatr Clin N Am 44 (2021) 393–403
https://doi.org/10.1016/j.psc.2021.04.010
0193-953X/21/© 2021 Elsevier Inc. All rights reserved.

nonathletes, athletes tend to sleep less per night and the quality of their sleep also remains lower.[2] This can be attributed to the high pressure of competitive environments combined with the disruption of circadian rhythms that surround training schedules, practice times, and travels across time zones. Left untreated, this can lead to the development of long-term mental health conditions, for example, depression, anxiety, and substance abuse. Furthermore, inadequate sleep among athletes may lead to a decline in physical performance (eg, speed, accuracy, reaction times, peak power output, endurance), decline in cognitive performance (eg, attention and memory), and an increase in the risk of illness and injury.

Adequate sleep involves consideration of its timing, quality, and quantity. A sleep duration of a minimum of 8 to 9 hours in a 24-hour period is typically needed, although this varies based on age, training (type, duration, intensity, timing), innate circadian rhythms, and health status. Population-based studies suggest that athletes on an average sleep less than the general population: The National Collegiate Athletic Association (NCAA) Inter-Association Task Force on Sleep and Wellness reports that in-season student-athletes average 6.27 hours of sleep nightly.[3] In a survey of 14,134 collegiate athletes at NCAA member institutions, 61% of student-athletes report daytime fatigue at least 3 or more days in a week; this could impact academic performance, sports performance, and overall wellness. In a 2018 single-institution study of 628 collegiate athletes from 29 varsity teams, 42% experienced poor sleep quality (measured by the Pittsburgh Sleep Quality Index [PSQI]) and 51% reported high levels of excessive daytime sleepiness (assessed by the Epworth Sleepiness Scale).[4] In the NCAA Growth, Opportunities, Aspirations, and Learning of Students survey study, less than 25% of collegiate athletes reported ≥ 8 hours of sleep on a typical night, and 70% of male and 82% of female collegiate athletes reported a preference for more sleep.[5]

Athletes are carefully monitored regarding their nutrition, physiologic and metabolic states, and parameters carefully followed as they relate to the impact on performance. Interestingly, sleep is often overlooked, and its relationship to overall performance is neglected. There is a growing awareness of the need to address this and to ensure that sleep health is integrated into the athletes' overall health maintenance strategy.

UNDERLYING FACTORS CONTRIBUTING TO SLEEP DISORDERS AMONG ATHLETES

Major determinants of the amount of sleep that an athlete may need include their chronotype, type of sport they are engaged in, and the type and timing of training. The chronotype or circadian rhythm is an internal process that regulates the sleep-wake cycle. Shifting the circadian rhythm is called entrainment. Morning or early chronotypes show better race times, show higher brain excitability in the morning, and perceive exercise to be harder in the evening.[6] In a small study by Tamm and colleagues, 18 participants (9 morning chronotypes and 9 evening chronotypes) were evaluated using magnetic stimulation of the cortex, and isometric torque measurements. Excitability of the motor cortex and the spinal cord, maximum oxygen uptake, and muscle torque and strength were greatest at the time correlated to their chronotype, that is, evening types performed at their peak in late in the day.[7]

It is unclear of the role played by lifestyle behaviors, including smoking, drinking, diet, and use of electronics, on sleep health in athletes; however, fundamental to addressing sleep disorders among athletes involves doing a comprehensive assessment of these factors in addition to other possible factors, including pain, mental health issues, including addiction-related issues, medications, central sleep apnea, and prior sports-related injuries, including concussions.

BARRIERS TO A COMPREHENSIVE APPROACH TO TREATING SLEEP DISORDERS IN ATHLETES

Clear communication of treatment and management strategies among all the members of a treatment team is essential to boosting the overall health and performance of athletes. **Table 1** presents factors that impact the collaborative approach to diagnosing and treating sleep disorders in athletes.

HOW DO SLEEP DISORDERS IMPACT MENTAL HEALTH?

There are no well-designed studies that look at sleep disorders and their impact on the mental health of an athlete. Patients in the general population with irregular sleep patterns or sleep disorders tend to have poor quality of life, poor response to treatments as well as high rates of relapse or remission of psychiatric disorders. There is evidence to suggest that long-term sleep disorders (primarily insomnia and sleep apnea) predispose patients to mental health disorders, including major depressive disorder, mania, generalized anxiety disorders (GAD), and substance abuse disorders. Insomnia/sleep disorders remain important diagnostic criteria for anxiety (almost 50% with GAD report sleep disturbances), posttraumatic stress disorder (PTSD) (in form of distressing dreams), and substance abuse disorders. Of note, in nonathlete populations, studies

Table 1	
Factors impacting diagnosing and treating sleep disorders	
Factors	**Comments**
Lack of education	Sleep disorders are not emphasized in medical school and specialty training curricula; for example, the *DSM-5* provides only a small section on sleep disorders
Limited awareness	Sleep advice to elite athletes from coaches, trainers, and medical staff is often limited to pamphlets on "sleep hygiene"
Treatment fragmentation	Elite athletes have access to a multidisciplinary team, but the emphasis on sleep remains limited
Inadequate research	There are almost no well-designed studies on sleep interventions for elite athletes
Generalization	The elite athlete is different than the general population and requires a targeted and a focused approach to sleep management
Sleep problem solving, rather than prevention	Athletes do not always advocate for themselves and seek help only when a problem manifests, sometimes because of underlying stigma and fear
Lack of specificity	Diagnosing and managing sleep disorders requires an understanding of the athletes physical and mental health
Competing priorities	Competing priorities, for example, training and competition schedules, social and media appearances, are often prioritized over sleep
Resources	Resource allocation to promote healthy sleep in athletes depends on needs of the team and other stakeholders (team owners, managers, investors, and so forth) who must be included in the process
Guidelines	There is a need for evidence-based guidelines to promote healthy sleep behaviors and associated interventions for athletes

have demonstrated that treatments to improve sleep in patients with PTSD (which include cognitive-behavioral therapy approaches for insomnia, hyperarousal, and sleep avoidance) can also improve PTSD symptoms.[8] Thus, it is important that sleep and mental health disorders are treated concurrently, to improve treatment outcomes.

THE IMPACT OF SLEEP PROBLEMS ON ATHLETIC PERFORMANCE

Sleep disturbances tend to impact overall health and may result in neurocognitive, metabolic, immunologic, and cardiovascular dysfunction. Sleep disturbances have been associated with adversely impacting peak power output, endurance, and reaction time. A systematic review of 48 studies by Wardle-Pinkston and colleagues[9] concluded that insomnia is associated with decreased attention and cognitive performance. Directly and indirectly, sleep problems may determine whether an athlete makes the team or not, is chosen for a tournament or is sidelined, remains injury free or is injured and has a prolonged rehabilitation phase, makes the podium or is dismissed, has a healthy career or has it cut short. In that an athlete's sports performance is so intrinsically linked to their identity, the impact of sleep as an overall predictor of their long-term mental health must be assessed.

THE APPROACH TO SLEEP PROBLEMS IN THE ATHLETE

The most commonly used tools to measure sleep disturbances in the general population include The Sleep Hygiene Index, Insomnia Severity Index, Epworth Sleepiness Scale, Morningness-Eveningness Questionnaire, and the PSQI. However, these have limited utility when it comes to sleep screening in the athlete population.[10] For example, the PSQI, which has been the primary questionnaire used to assess sleep in athletes, has not been validated in an athlete population, is difficult to score, lacks information specific to athletes, and shows poor concordance rates with the clinical assessment of a sleep medicine physician.

The Athlete Sleep Screening Questionnaire (ASSQ) and Athlete Sleep Behavior Questionnaire (ASBQ) have been studied, validated, and specifically designed for the athlete population. The ASBQ was developed by Matthew Driller and colleagues and consists of an 18-item questionnaire to identify faulty sleep behaviors in athletes, rather than sleep disorders.[10] It helps determine which athletes would benefit from preventive measures and which athletes suffer from significant sleep problems. The ASSQ was developed by Dr Charles Samuels and his colleagues,[11] it consists of 15 items, is reliable and consistent, and is an excellent tool to screen athletes for sleep problems (**Table 2**).

The ASSQ and ASBQ are used to guide the formulation of the athlete' sleep optimization strategy, which may include sleep coaching, cognitive behavioral therapy, sleep medicine consultation, and or medication.

TREATING ATHLETES FOR COMORBID DISORDERS

Sleep management requires a coordinated approach by the athlete's multidisciplinary team (**Table 3**).

Tools and interventions should be made available to not just normalize the athletes sleep but also optimize it. **Fig. 1** provides a schema, *The Pyramid of Peak Sleep Performance*, that is used in the authors' practice when working with elite athletes in professional sports. The approach is to use the evidence in the existing literature and apply those strategies to the sleep of the athlete, providing a systematic mitigation strategy to address the multifactorial issues related to the sleep disorder.

Table 2
The Athlete Sleep Behavior Questionnaire for screening athletes for sleep problems

No.	In Recent Times (over the Last Month)	Never	Rarely	Sometimes	Frequently	Always
1	I take afternoon naps lasting 2 or more hours					
2	I use stimulants when I train/ compete (eg, caffeine)					
3	I exercise (train or compete) late at night (after 7 PM)					
4	I consume alcohol within 4 h of going to bed					
5	I go to bed at different times each night (more than ±1 h variation)					
6	I go to bed feeling thirsty					
7	I go to bed with sore muscles					
8	I use light-emitting technology in the hour leading up to bedtime (eg, laptop, phone, television, video games)					
9	I think, plan, and worry about my sporting performance when I am in bed					
10	I think, plan, and worry about issues not related to my sport when I am in bed					
11	I use sleeping pills/tablets to help me sleep					
12	I wake to go to the bathroom more than once per night					
13	I wake myself and/or my bed partner with my snoring					
14	I wake myself and/or my bed partner with my muscle twitching					
15	I get up at different times each morning (more than ±1 h variation)					
16	At home, I sleep in a less than ideal environment (eg, too light, too noisy, uncomfortable bed/pillow, too hot/cold)					
17	I sleep in foreign environments (eg, hotel rooms)					
18	Travel gets in the way of building a consistent sleep-wake routine					

Scoring:
Never = 1, Rarely = 2, Sometimes = 3, Frequently = 4, Always = 5

Total Global Score: _____

Table 3
The sleep health team

Professional	Role
Sleep medicine physician	Helps guide diagnostic and treatment strategies
Sport Psychiatrist	Collaborates with the sleep specialist on the best psychotherapeutic and psychopharmacologic interventions
Team doctor	Administers sleep screening tools (ASSQ and ABSQ), and diagnostic workups and specialty consultations
Nutritionist	Reinforces sleep education, collaborates with team to design meal plans to promote sleep health
Coaches	Reinforce sleep education in athletes with an emphasis on performance optimization
Trainers	Reinforce sleep education in athletes with an emphasis on physical performance metrics, collaborate with sleep medicine (timing of training, chronotype, strategic napping, and so forth)
Physical therapists/rehabilitation	Reinforce sleep education in athletes with an emphasis on risk of injury, rehabilitation, and return to play
Athletic directors	Collaborate with the team on preseason, in-season, and off-season schedules. Discuss the best means, timing, and duration of transportation, training, and other logistical aspects of sleep
Sports psychologist	Reinforce sleep education in athletes with an emphasis on mental resilience, both measurements and tracking improvements

The current sleep guidelines from the American Academy of Sleep Medicine do not have separate guidelines for athletes at this point in time. Thus, the treatment of sleep breathing disorders, parasomnias, sleep movement disorders, circadian rhythm disorders, and hypersomnias in athletes are the same as the general population. Insomnia is by far the most commonly encountered sleep disorder in athletes, and so the authors address the best treatment approaches to insomnia in the athlete.

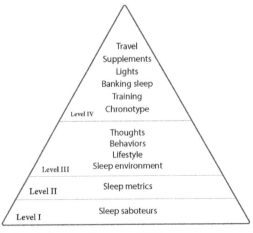

Fig. 1. The pyramid of peak sleep performance (PSP).

INSOMNIA TREATMENT
Cognitive Behavioral Therapy for Insomnia

The key sleep strategies for insomnia are rooted in Cognitive Behavioral Therapy for Insomnia (CBT-I) (**Box 1**). CBT-I is a multicomponent treatment that addresses patients' cognitions and behaviors that interfere with sleep. A meta-analysis of 30 randomized controlled trials comparing CBT-I with nonactive control groups in the general population demonstrated that CBT-I produces clinically significant effects that last up to a year after therapy.[12]

Arthur Spielman created a conceptual model of primary insomnia that identifies *predisposing factors, precipitating events, and perpetuating mechanisms* that contribute to the development and maintenance of chronic insomnia. According to this model, some individuals may be particularly vulnerable, or *predisposed*, to sleep problems by virtue of having a "highly sensitive" or "malfunctioning" biological sleep system or a hyperactive arousal system that interferes with sleep. In individuals with a *predisposition* for insomnia, disruptive circumstances, such as stressful life events, often *precipitate* sleep difficulties. In individuals who are not predisposed to insomnia, stress-induced sleep problems are usually transient and resolve when the original distress subsides. However, according to this model, some people become overly focused on their sleep problems. This focus tends to *perpetuate* their sleep difficulties because it can produce heightened anxiety about sleep and the development of maladaptive strategies and practices that, although intended to improve sleep, actually worsen it.

Maladaptive strategies include *avoidance behaviors* during waking hours. Avoidance behaviors may include canceling planned activities, either because of feeling too tired or due to fear that such activities will interfere with sleep, spending excessive time in bed, and developing rigid sleep-related rituals. These behaviors are manifestations of increased *sleep effort*. Simply stated, the individual is *trying too hard* to sleep. In response to poor sleep, *sleep-interfering thoughts* may develop that include overestimating and worrying about the negative consequences of poor sleep and approaching bedtime with fear of failure. Behavioral and cognitive responses to sleep problems, and some of the practices for coping with them, create a vicious cycle by prolonging or worsening the very problems they are trying to solve.

Box 1
Cognitive-behavioral therapy for insomnia

1. An important component of CBT-I is education regarding the processes that regulates sleep.

2. The *behavioral component* includes stimulus control and sleep restriction therapy.
   a. Stimulus control works through the extinction of a *conditioned arousal* (patients' beds and bedrooms have become associated with wakefulness and an inability to let go, relax, and fall asleep).
   b. Sleep restriction therapy works by initially reducing the amount of time the individual spends in bed in order to build up pressure for sleep.

3. The *cognitive component* of CBT-I is based on the theory that a person's beliefs and the manner in which he thinks about, perceives, interprets, or assigns judgment to particular situations in his life affects his emotional experiences.

4. The final component of CBT-I aims to reduce *physiologic hyperarousal,* defined as high activity in the sympathetic nervous system, and *cognitive hyperarousal.* Training in relaxation techniques, implementing a *scheduled worry time,* creating a time to unwind before sleep, and using cognitive therapy strategies.

Sleep Supplements

Melatonin is the most widely studied sleep supplement in the general population. There are other supplements used to treat insomnia (**Box 2**). However, rigorous studies looking at the efficacy of these supplements on the athlete population (for sleep improvement as well as athletic performance correlations) are lacking.

Exercise Interventions

Altering the athlete's academic and training schedules around an extended sleeping period remains vital to achieving a balanced internal homeostasis.[15] Exercise tends to suppress secretion of melatonin, boosts neurotransmitters like adrenaline and dopamine, and thus may contribute to sleep disruptions if it is done too close to bedtime. The existing literature suggests that training and sleep schedules should be tailored based on the athlete's profile:

- The timing of training has a direct effect on sports performance.
- Evening or afternoon training contributes to better sports performance in intermediate chronotypes and late chronotypes.
- Morning chronotypes may benefit when training and competition is scheduled early.
- Reduced sleep quality following evening training sessions may negatively impact subsequent performance in morning chronotypes.

IMPACT OF SLEEP OPTIMIZATION ON PERFORMANCE OUTCOMES

When designing a health maintenance plan, consideration should be given to a composite of factors, including the athletes physical and mental health; lifestyle factors

---

Box 2
Sleep supplements

1. Melatonin is used as a sleep aid and also is purported to have anti-inflammatory and antioxidant properties. Its best use is to help adjust to a different time zone, along with travel strategies such as strategic napping and light blocking (expanded on in later discussion).

2. Gamma butyric acid (GABA) is an inhibitory neurotransmitter and suppresses the excitatory neurotransmitters norepinephrine and glutamate. It may facilitate onset and duration of sleep.

This combination may be useful for initial insomnia or difficulty falling asleep.

3. L-Theanine increases the production of dopamine, serotonin, and GABA, all of which may promote sleep and elevate mood. It may improve sleep quality, overall sleep time and reduced anxiety, nightmares, and improved overall energy in patients with attention-deficit/hyperactivity disorder.[13]

4. Passionflower may boost the level of GABA in the brain to enhance sleep in patients with insomnia.

5. Magnesium deficiency can result in neural overexcitation causing anxiety, restlessness, and sleep problems. One study measured hormonal and electrical changes in the brain of older persons during sleep and found that magnesium supplementation improved both hormonal and electrical patterns in the brain during sleep.[14]

6. Chamomile is rich in a flavonoid called apigenin that binds to benzodiazepine receptors in the brain. Potential benefits include improvements in sleep latency, nighttime awakenings, daytime functioning, and fatigue severity.

7. Valerian root, lemon balm extract, vitamin B6, and 5-HTP are other candidates to manage insomnia, although no good data exist to support their use.

Box 3
Recommendations for interventions to improve sleep health in the athlete

1. Ensure that sleep health is assessed in athletes, that sleep screening tools designed for athletes are used, and that consultation with a sleep specialist is available when indicated.

2. Provide dedicated educational/sleep training programs to not just simply screen athletes for sleep disorders but also give *specific* guidance on sleep optimization.

3. Have trainers, coaches, and data scientists use performance metrics to monitor how specific sleep interventions impact sports performance.

4. Consult with a sleep medicine specialist with expertise in sports on ways to promote sleep health of the team.

(sleep environment, nutrition, stressors, social engagements, and so forth); chronotype; sleep needs (quantity of sleep typically required for peak performance); competition times and travel. For example, traveling westward has been shown to worsen performance; NBA teams that traveled eastward scored more points per game and had a winning percentage of 45.4% compared with 36.2% for teams. There is a need to restore natural sleep patterns in between busy schedules and travels of athletes to ensure that internal homeostasis remains balanced, helping athletes feel less fatigue and sleepiness during wakeful hours. If athletes are trained to adjust their sleep patterns, their cognitive performance, reaction times, psychomotor vigilance tasks, alertness, vigor, and mood can all improve.

Sleep extension and strategic napping remain other alternate mechanisms that can be taught to athletes. Preliminary studies have shown that sleep extension in athletes can help improve performance.

Research on sleep extension in athletes is still in the early stages, and research is needed to investigate the performance benefits using defined outcome measures. In a systematic review of 10 studies comprising a total of 218 athletes in the age range of 18 to 24 years from various sports (eg, swimming, soccer, basketball, tennis), it was reported that sleep extension had the most beneficial effects on subsequent performance (compared with napping, sleep hygiene, and postexercise recovery strategies).[15] Strategic napping is a way of using naps at certain intervals, based on total sleep need, chronotype, time of competition, and time zone, in order to enhance recovery and performance. Preliminary evaluations suggest a performance benefit, although once again more study is needed.[16,17] **Box 3** provides recommendations

---

Box 4
Future directions to determine the impact of sleep on sports performance

1. There needs to be specific research that looks at the bidirectional relationship of sleep problems and specific mental health problems, as well as the impact of psychotropic medications on sleep and sports performance, in athletes.

2. There is a great need for more research on the impact of CBT-I on sleep in athletes.

3. Each player should be monitored with questionnaires such as the Acute Recovery and Stress Scale and the REST-Q Sport to measure self-perceived travel fatigue, as well as ASSQ and ASBQ, sleep diaries, and other tools to correlate sleep disruptions with mental health and performance outcomes.

4. A personalized medicine approach, including biomarker assessments, to the health management of athletes may provide guidance on how to maximize performance.

on interventions to improve sleep health, and **Box 4** provides recommendations for future research in improving sleep health in athletes.

SUMMARY

Considering the complexities of sleep problems and comorbid psychiatric issues, as well as the direct impact on sports performance, there is a benefit to prioritizing sleep health in the athlete. In recent years, there has been an increase in awareness of these benefits, although well-designed research is needed to validate their impact. In addition to educational interventions, there is a need to identify best practice strategies and disseminate them through professional guidelines. If athlete health and sleep are considered the priority, everybody wins. It will allow for record-shattering performances, less injuries, longer playing careers, and happier teams, players, fans, and sponsors.

DISCLOSURE

S.A. Creado: Earnings from Amen Clinics, Inc and Shane Creado, LLC. Royalties from BrainMD, Inc, Amen University, Amazon, Inc. S. Advani: No disclosures.

REFERENCES

1. Roth T, Coulouvrat C, Hajak G, et al. Prevalence and perceived health associated with insomnia based on DSM-IV-TR; International Statistical Classification of Diseases and Related Health Problems, Tenth Revision; and Research Diagnostic Criteria/International Classification of Sleep Disorders, Second Edition criteria: results from the America Insomnia Survey. Biol Psychiatry 2011;69(6):592–600.
2. Simpson N, Gibbs E, Maheson G. Optimizing sleep to maximize performance: implications and recommendation for elite athletes. Scand J Med Sci Sports 2017;27:266–74.
3. Kroshus E, Wagner J, Wyrick D, et al. Wake up call for collegiate athlete sleep: narrative review and consensus recommendations from the NCAA Interassociation Task Force on Sleep and Wellness. Br J Sports Med 2019;53(12):731–6.
4. Mah CD, Kezirian EJ, Marcello BM, et al. Poor sleep quality and insufficient sleep of a collegiate student-athlete population. Sleep Health 2018;4:251–7.
5. National Collegiate Athletic Association. NCAA GOALS study. Indianapolis, IN: National Collegiate Athletic Association; 2016. Available at: http://www.ncaa. org/about/resources/research/ncaa-goals-study.
6. Laura C Rode.
7. Rudner TD, Rae DE. Impact of chronotype on athletic performance: current perspectives. ChronoPhysiol Ther 2017;7:1–6.
8. Tamm A, Lagerquist O, Ley A. Chronotype influences diurnal variations in the excitability of the human motor cortex and ability to generate torque during a maximum voluntary contraction. J Biolog Rhythms 2009;24:175–82.
9. Pollack MH, Hoge EA, Worthington JJ, et al. Eszopiclone for the treatment of posttraumatic stress disorder and associated insomnia: a randomized, double-blind, placebo-controlled trial. J Clin Psychiatry 2011;72(7):892–7.
10. Wardle-Pinkston S, Slavish DC, Taylor DJ. Insomnia and cognitive performance: a systematic review and meta-analysis. Sleep Med Rev 2019;48:101205.
11. Driller M, Mah C, Halson S. Development of the Athlete Sleep Behavior Questionnaire: a tool for identifying maladaptive sleep practices in elite athletes. Sleep Sci 2018;11(1):37–44.

12. Samuels C, James L, Lawson D, et al. The Athlete Sleep Screening Question-naire: a new tool for assessing and managing sleep in elite athletes. Br J Sports Med 2016;50(7):418–22.
13. der Zweerde T, Bisdounis L, Kyle S, et al. Cognitive behavioral therapy for insomnia: a meta-analysis of long-term effects in controlled studies. Sleep Med Rev 2019;48:101208.
14. Lyon M, Kapoor M, Juneja L. The effects of L-theanine (Suntheanine®) on objec-tive sleep quality in boys with attention deficit hyperactivity disorder (ADHD): a randomized, double-blind, placebo-controlled clinical trial. Altern Med Rev 2011;16:348–54.
15. Behnood A, et al. The effect of magnesium supplementation on primary insomnia in elderly: a double-blind placebo-controlled clinical trial. J Res Med Sci 2012; 17(12):1161–9.
16. Vitale JA, Weydahl A. Chronotype, physical activity, and sport performance: a systematic review. Sports Med 2017;47(9):1859–68.
17. Bonnar D, Bartel K, Kakoschke N, et al. Sleep interventions designed to improve athletic performance and recovery: a systematic review of current approaches. Sports Med 2018;48(3):683–703.

Substance Use and Its Impact on Athlete Health and Performance

Todd Stull, MD[a],*, Eric Morse, MD[b], David R. McDuff, MD[c,d]

KEYWORDS

- Anabolic • Doping • Alcohol • Stimulants • Opioids • Cannabis
- Performance enhancing

KEY POINTS

- Anabolic androgenic agents continue to be among the most common performance-enhancing agents used. Selective androgen receptor modulators are emerging as a class.
- Peptides, hormones, and metabolic modulators continue to be used and abused.
- Gene doping is in its early stages and continues to evolve.
- Detection methods continue to improve using biological passports.
- Alcohol misuse (i.e. binge drinking) remains common and can lead to a range of psychosocial, medical, and performance problems.
- Although the studies generally are of low quality; most conclude that the most common cannabinoids (ie, delta-9-tetrahydrocannabinol and cannabidiol) are not performance enhancing and more likely performance reducing.
- Many stimulants (eg, caffeine, methylphenidate/amphetamines, and ephedrine) are performance enhancing for indirect exercises measures of sports performance and may have serious side effects if used in high dosages or together (ie, stacked).

INTRODUCTION

Substance use has occurred through the ages to enhance performance, manage pain, and accelerate recovery. Doping is the use of a banned substance to improve athletic performance and is not restricted to elite athletes. Performance-enhancing substances can be illicit drugs or prescription medications or found in a variety of over-the-counter compounds or supplements. The present-day athlete who is seeking performance enhancement may use androgens (hormones), metabolic agents,

a Department of Psychiatry and Neuroscience, University of California, Riverside School of Medicine, Riverside, CA 92521, USA; b Carolina Performance, AIHF, 8300 Health Park #201, Raleigh, NC 27615, USA; c University of Maryland School of Medicine, Baltimore, MD, USA; d Maryland Centers for Psychiatry, 3290 North Ridge Road, Suite 320, Ellicott City, MD 21043, USA
* Corresponding author.
E-mail address: Todd.stull@ucr.edu

Psychiatr Clin N Am 44 (2021) 405–417
https://doi.org/10.1016/j.psc.2021.04.006
0193-953X/21/© 2021 Elsevier Inc. All rights reserved.

stimulants, opioids, anti-inflammatory agents, or endurance builders. *Ergogenic* and *ergolytic* are terms that refer to performance enhancement and performance impairment, respectively. In this review article the substances or methods used will cover the performance enhancing effects (ergogenic) and the performance impairing effects (ergolytic). **Box 1** summarizes the performance-enhancing substances and methods.

Despite risks, including medical complications, sanctions, and being banned from competition, athletes continue to seek out strategies to enhance performance. As a result of a series of scandals in international cycling, the World Anti-Doping Agency (WADA) was created in 1999 to address doping concerns and has developed accredited laboratories in addition to expanding testing procedures. Adverse Analytical Findings (AAFs) is a report from a WADA-approved laboratory that identifies the presence of a prohibited substance or its metabolites or markers or evidence of the use of a prohibited method. AAFs from 2003 to 2015 show that the 3 top substances identified were anabolic agents, stimulants, and diuretics. The WADA Code/Prohibited List is updated annually and is designed is to promote fair and ethical competition (**Box 2**).

ALCOHOL

Alcohol is legal, socially acceptable, consumed by fans, and advertised during sporting events and often part of team building and hazing. Athletes at all competitive levels use alcohol more commonly than any other substance except caffeine.

Prevalence/Reasons for Use

The prevalence of alcohol use in US professional sports largely is unknown due to privacy and negotiated collective bargaining agreements. According to the National Collegiate Athletic Association (NCAA), in 2017, 77% of student-athletes reported drinking alcohol in the past year, which is similar to the general population. Although 36% of student-athletes reported drinking on a weekly basis, approximately 2% reported drinking daily, and 42% of all student-athletes said they engage in binge drinking (4 or more drinks for women; 5 or more drinks for men in 1 sitting).[1]

Short-term and Long-term Side Effects/Reasons for Limiting/Quitting

Other than to reduce performance anxiety, alcohol sometimes is used to calm down from "stimulant stacking" in "upper-downer" pairings. The short-term effects of alcohol on performance physiology are more performance impairing than enhancing, in that they reduce balance, coordination, judgment, reasoning, and emotional control.

Box 1
Performance-enhancing substances and methods

- Mass builders—enhance strength, power, and explosiveness
- Endurance builders—improve the oxygen-carrying capacity
- Recovery enhancers—augment recovery and return to play/competition
- Inflammation and pain modulators
- Attention/alertness enhancers
- Blood manipulators
- Gene/cell modifiers

> **Box 2**
> **Types of antidoping rules violations**
>
> - Presence of prohibited substance or its metabolites in an athlete's sample
> - Use or attempted use of a prohibited substance or method
> - Refusing or failing without justification to submit sample
> - Whereabouts violations
> - Tampering or attempted tampering with any part of doping control
> - Possession of prohibited substances or methods
> - Trafficking or attempted trafficking in any prohibited substances or method
> - Administration or attempted administration of any prohibited method or substance or assisting, encouraging, aiding, abetting, and covering up

In the long term, alcohol misuse may lead to depression, anxiety, loss of libido, and reduced socialization. The consequences of use and the recommendations of treatment professionals often lead to reduction or cessation of alcohol use, for example, legal problems and injury. Injury rates more than double when athletes drink at least weekly versus nondrinkers; athletes who drink to cope have more negative consequences than those who drink for other reasons.

Although alcohol use first may be recognized during urine drug testing (an alcohol screen detects alcohol consumption only within 4–6 hours before a test whereas Liquid chromatography mass spectrometry (LCMS) or gas chromatography mass spectrometry (GCMS) tests for ethyl glucuronide or ethylsulfate detect alcohol consumption out to 80 hours). The most efficient way to assess alcohol use is to ask how much and how often, as opposed to a simple, "Do you or don't you?" In addition, clinicians experienced with substance use disorders generally are more adept at recognizing the subtle signs and symptoms of use (**Table 1**).

Effects on Performance

Alcohol negatively effects performance, reducing aerobic performance and delivering empty calories that may cause weight gain with reduced muscle mass, and associated hangovers that interfere with practice or performance. In 2018, WADA removed alcohol from the air sports, automobile, archery, and powerboating prohibited list.[2] The World Archery Federation put out a statement against its removal on October 1, 2017, claiming studies in the 1980s did show alcohol is performance enhancing. Alcohol remains on the NCAA prohibited list for rifle in that small amounts may lower heart rates because rifle athletes aim to pull the trigger between beats.

In summary, alcohol continues to have widespread use among athletes despite the negative effects on performance and health. Different effects occur with short-term and long-term use on health and performance.

ANDROGENS

Anabolic androgenic steroids (AASs) make up half of all AAFs in drug testing from WADA laboratories. Recent results from WADA laboratories indicate selective androgen receptor modulators (SARMs), such as MK-2866, RAD-140, and LGD-4033, are becoming increasingly popular.[2]

SARMs are a class of nonsteroidal androgen receptor ligands that bind to tissue specific areas. They promote transcription and regulation of gene expression and have an

Table 1
Recognition of substance use and abuse

Substance	Signs and Symptoms of Use	Signs and Symptoms of Withdrawal
Stimulant	Dilated pupils, anxiety, jitteriness, increased heart rate/blood pressure, dry mouth, nasal problems, restlessness, insomnia, talkativeness, loss of appetite, tics	Fatigue, headaches, anxiety, depression somnolence
Cannabis	Smell on clothes, bloodshot eyes, memory problems, lack of motivation, paranoia, increased appetite, use of eyedrops, drowsiness, slowed responses, cough	Insomnia, cravings, irritability anxiety, reduced appetite
Alcohol	Sedation, disinhibition, slurred speech euphoria, ataxia, blackouts, memory problems, flushing, impulsiveness vomiting, fights, legal problems, sweating	Increased heart rate/blood pressure, tremor, seizures, irritability, insomnia fatigue, depressed mood, headache, nystagmus
Anabolic steroids	Men-reduced testicular size, low sperm count, balding, Prostate cancer risk, Painful urination, Breast development (irreversible except through plastic surgery), Infertility. Women-facial hair, voice deepening, baldness, Enlarged clitoris, Menstrual dysfunction. Both Genders-weight increase, oily hair/skin, Cysts, High cholesterol & blood pressure, Heightened sexual desire, Acne, Shaking, Behavioral changes (aggressiveness), Stretch marks, bloating.	Depressed mood, weakness, fatigue, aches, insomnia, weight loss, restlessness, insomnia, mood swings
Opioids	Constricted pupils, sedation, euphoria, track marks, confusion, less pain, constipation	Muscle aches, restlessness, insomnia, enlarged pupils, rhinorrhea, diarrhea, stomach and leg cramps, goose flesh, sweats, nausea

anabolic effect on skeletal muscle and bone. A perceived advantage of using SARMs is the anabolic effects of increasing muscle mass and power, while not getting the undesired androgenic effects, such as hirsutism, clitoromegaly, and gynecomastia. AASs bind with the androgen receptor and via DNA binding-dependent manner to regulate gene transcription, or in a non–DNA-binding–dependent manner to influence cellular activity or through ligand-independent actions of the androgen receptor. There is a steroid response element on the DNA that becomes gene activated and promotes transcription and then translation to produce proteins and muscle hypertrophy. This increased muscle mass enhances power, strength, and ultimately performance. Recent data suggest that the performance-enhancing effects of AASs last much longer that the period of administration and the myonuclei numbers are not lost after abstinence.[3]

Direct doping involves administration of endogenous or synthetic androgens. Indirect doping refers to administration of nonandrogenic drugs that increase endogenous testosterone to gain a performance advantage. This includes the use of human chorionic gonadotropin and luteinizing hormone (LH), antiestrogens, including estrogen receptor antagonist or inhibitors. Natural androgen precursors like dehydroepiandrosterone or androstenedione are converted to testosterone or dihydrotestosterone or epitestosterone and are used to mask the testosterone/epitestosterone (T/E) ratio that is used for detection in drug testing. Athletes unwillingly may ingest ergogenic substances by taking over-the-counter dietary supplements that may contain amphetamines, AASs, SARMs, growth factors, prohormones, and erythropoietin (EPO).

PEPTIDE HORMONES, GROWTH FACTORS, RELATED SUBSTANCES, AND MIMETICS

Hemoglobin mass is an important component to influence aerobic power. The erythropoiesis-stimulating agents include EPO, a glycoprotein, which increases oxygen supply to muscle and increase endurance and enhancing performance via proliferation of red blood cells. EPO production can be activated by hypoxia-inducible factors (HIFs).

HIFs are cell-based substances that make EPO. The uses of HIFs are pharmacologic and/or genetic strategies that activate the effects of hypoxia to increase EPO to stimulate red blood cell production and delivery of oxygen to tissues.

Growth hormone (GH) and related factors and secretagogues aim to stimulate endogenous GH secretion to enhance the GH/insulinlike growth factor (IGF)-1 relationship. Several factors regulate GH production. GH stimulates the release IGF-1 and IGF-2. The effects of GH are mediated through IGF-1. There is a noted decrease in fat mass and an increase in lean body mass and bone mineral density. It increases protein synthesis, bone growth and density, muscle mass, strength, maximal oxygen uptake, maximal heart rate, and power output. IGF-1 increases Vo_2 max, insulin sensitivity in skeletal muscle, protein synthesis, bone growth, and fat metabolism.

HORMONE AND METABOLIC MODULATORS

Hormone and metabolic modulators are a group of synthetic compounds that regulate endogenous hormones and muscle pathways that enhance performance or to counteract the side effects of other agents. The AASs have anabolic effects and inhibit the release of gonadotropin-releasing hormone, follicle-stimulating hormone, and LH, and this results in a hypogonadotropic state and decreases testosterone levels. The use of an antiestrogenic substance in sports can mitigate this antiestrogen effect. The aromatase inhibitors limit the conversion of testosterone to estrogen, thereby increasing testosterone and androstenedione levels and promoting anabolic effects. This group includes both steroidal and nonsteroidal substances. They may be beneficial in men to diminish the unwanted side effects of AASs. The selective estrogen receptor modulators (SERMs) target specific tissues and have the potential to elevate testosterone. SERMs mainly are used to treat the side effects of AASs. Negative regulation of skeletal muscle through activin type II transmembrane receptors can decrease muscle mass. Myostatin is a key regulator of muscle mass and function and is a myokine that diminishes muscle growth. Myostatin inhibitors lead to muscle hyperplasia and hypertrophy. Agents affecting transforming growth factor that influence activin IIB receptors possess the potential to enhance performance in sports by increasing muscle mass.

Metabolic modulators are a class of substances where the mechanism of action is focused on regulation of metabolic pathways and include peroxisome proliferator-activated receptor-delta (PPARd), agonist-GW1516, GW1516, adenosine monophosphate–activated protein kinase (AMPK), insulin and insulin-mimetics, and meldonium. PPARd has multiple metabolic effects and agonists exert their effects on the muscle fiber. These include elevated fatty acid oxidation, reduced obesity and insulin resistance, exercise-induced muscle remodeling, and increased performance. Shifting of substrate utilization, preservation of glucose, and influence on mitochondrial machinery prolong performance.[4] Another example, GW501516, shifts metabolism from carbohydrates to fat in skeletal muscle. AMPK and meldonium have anti-ischemic effects and appear cardioprotective. AMPK can regulate glucose and lipid metabolism and therefore energy use. Meldonium appears to reduce oxygen use during exercise.

Prevalence/Reasons for Use

Data from WADA laboratories reported the most common AAFs in all sports between 2013 and 2017 were anabolic agents. Despite the WADA laboratories' results indicating that most positive results are androgens, the anabolic agents, including SARMs, continue to increase. Hormone and metabolic modulators are increasing as well, especially GW1516, in the past 2 years. The NCAA reports the use of anabolic steroids in 2009, 2013, and 2017 at 0.4% when averaging the data for all men's and women's sports.

Low-concentration positive tests of anabolic agents, such as Turinabol, clenbuterol, and stanozolol, along with the SARMs ostarine, RAD-140, and LGD-4033 and the hormone and metabolic modulatory GW1116 are being detected more frequently. This may be from the use of supplements or possibly microdosing. Microdosing is the use of small, frequents amounts of a substance to avoid detection yet benefit from the performance-enhancing effects. The goal is to gain a performance advantage while trying to stay below the detection threshold. The prevalence rates of microdosing are unknown.

Short-Term and Long-Term Side Effects/Reasons for Limiting/Quitting

Signs and symptoms of use and withdrawal related to AASs can effect many organ systems, including cardiovascular, psychiatric, reproductive, musculoskeletal, renal, immune, inflammatory and hypothalamic-pituitary-testicular axis, and are well documented in the literature (see **Box 2**).

Effects on Performance

Numerous studies support the ergogenic effects of AASs. They increase muscle mass, strength, power, explosiveness, endurance, fat loss, muscle recovery, aggression, motivation, and hemoglobin to improve oxygen carrying capacity.[5]

In summary, AASs continue to be the most common doping method, and use is increasing. Methods to enhance performance, such as gene modification and use of transcription factors to influence protein synthesis, along with microdosing are emerging strategies. The challenge remains for testing to keep up with innovations in formulation and delivery. The hematological and steroidal Athlete Biological Passport (ABP) is being used more in the testing process and the endocrine model soon may be available.

OPIOIDS

The opioid epidemic has affected the prescribing habits of all physicians, including those in sports medicine. In the late 1990s, physicians were encouraged to treat pain aggressively as the "fifth vital sign" and were told that oxycodone was not addictive. The pendulum has swung back to reduce the prescribing of opioids and encourage the prescribing of nonopioid pain relievers; this is relevant particularly to subacute and long-term management.

Prevalence/Reasons for Use

According to a 2017 NCAA report, 11% of student-athletes use narcotic pain medication with a prescription, down from 18% in 2013; 3% of student-athletes reported using narcotic pain medication without a prescription in the past year, less than the general US population, ages 18 to 25, of 5.6%; 2% of student-athletes reported misusing narcotic pain medication. Rates of past year use/misuse of nonprescription opioids are higher among male athletes and female collegiate athletes than nonathletes (18% for male athletes and 11% for female athletes), especially in power, collision, and higher injury frequency sports like football and wrestling.[6]

The prevalence of opioid use in professional sports largely is unknown due to privacy and negotiated collective bargaining agreements. One National Institute of Drug Abuse study of 644 former National Football League (NFL) players found that 52% used pain medication while playing.[7] Of that 52%, 63% obtained the medication from a nonmedical source and 15% still were misusing pain medication. A follow-up study 9 years later showed that 50% of those former NFL players still were using opioids. The leading associated risk factors were risky drinking and opioid use during NFL careers to relieve stress or relax.

The reasons for opioid use are similar to those for other substances (eg, socialization, feel good, coping, and performance), but they are used most frequently for relieving pain.

Short-Term and Long-Term Side Effects/Reasons for Limiting/Quitting

Opioid use in the short term may help with acute pain, energy, motivation, and mood and produce a sense of well-being. Side effects and withdrawal symptoms are included in **Box 2**. Long-term side effects include use disorder, overdose, abnormal pain sensitivity, low testosterone and reduced energy, drive, mood, sleep quality, libido, and fertility.

Effects of Performance

According to the WADA 2020 Prohibited List of Substances, certain opioids are prohibited in-competition. Use of these narcotics in-competition requires an approved therapeutic use exception. Codeine, hydrocodone, and tramadol are in the Monitoring Program and currently are permitted. There currently is no literature on the performance-enhancing effects of these substances; however, it is felt that these substances enhance performance through blocking the body's pain signals.

STIMULANTS

Stimulants (uppers) are a broad class of substances that primarily activate (or inhibit) brain circuits that use epinephrine, dopamine, norepinephrine, nicotine-acetylcholine, and adenosine (inhibition) as well as the sympathetic nervous system. This class includes legal stimulants (eg, caffeine, nicotine, and cathinone-khat), illicit stimulants (eg, cocaine, methamphetamine, and methylenedioxymethamphetamine), prescribed medications (eg, methylphenidate, amphetamine, modafinil, phentermine, and bupropion), and over-the-counter medications or supplements (eg, ephedrine, pseudoephedrine, and synephrine). They can be used recreationally/socially, as performance enhancers, or both. Most members of this class are banned or limited by the WADA, US Professional sports leagues, and the NCAA because of their known performance-enhancing effects.[8] When prescribed clinically, they can be used to treat attention-deficit/hyperactivity disorder (ADHD), excessive daytime sleepiness, narcolepsy, depression, and obesity. If prescribed by a licensed physician for certain conditions (eg, ADHD and narcolepsy), they can be used after obtaining a therapeutic use or medical exemption.

Prevalence/Reasons for Use

Caffeine currently is the most widely used stimulant by elite athletes, especially at international and Olympic levels. Following its removal from the WADA prohibited substances list in 2004 and its inclusion in the monitoring program, urine testing showed that caffeine was detected in competition in 70% of Spanish Olympic sports competitors; the sports with the highest concentrations were cycling, rowing, triathlon, and track and field.[9] Caffeine use is attractive across many sports because its ingestion in tablets, gels, liquids, or supplements both before and during competition increases alertness, vigilance, muscle endurance, muscle strength, anaerobic power, and aerobic endurance.

Nicotine is the second most widely used stimulant in elite sports. Its use is common especially in US collegiate and professional lacrosse, ice hockey, and baseball. Use includes cigars, spit tobacco, hookahs, cigarettes, and e-cigarettes. Nicotine can be obtained via oral tobacco use, smoking, or vaping. It is attractive because of its perceived effects to increase alertness, concentration, memory, focus, energy, and endurance; produce relaxation and calmness; and reduce boredom.

Prescribed stimulants for ADHD appear to be the third most widely used stimulant in sports. The NCAA reports that 5% of all student athletes use either methylphenidate or amphetamine formulations without a prescription, whereas an additional 7% use with a prescription.[10] Major League Baseball is the only US professional sports that reports its therapeutic use exemptions for ADHD annually; in 2018, they reported that approximately 8.4% of its 40-man roster players were approved to use prescription stimulants.[11] Prescribed stimulants are used with or without a prescription to increase alertness, reduce distractibility, combat fatigue, boost energy, improve reaction time, enhance focus and sustained attention, and reduce hyperactivity and impulsivity.

The use of readily available illicit stimulants like cocaine, methamphetamine, and 3,4-methylenedioxymethamphetamine (MDMA) appear similar in elite athletes to that in the general population. Cocaine is used recreationally for its euphoric and energizing effects and often is used concurrently with alcohol. It can be sniffed intranasally, smoked or dissolved in water, and injected. It has high rates for the development of a use disorder and some serious short-term side effects, for example, anxiety, paranoia, and irregular or rapid heat rate.

Over-the-counter stimulants like ephedra/ephedrine and synephrine, are found primarily in supplements that are advertised to help athletes boost exercise intensity and/or to lose weight. They often are combined with caffeine compounding the stimulant effect. Ephedrine was banned by the Food and Drug Administration in 2004 following the heat stroke death of a Major League Baseball player in 2003 and a subsequent analyses of serious incident reports indicating higher rates of heart attack, seizure, stroke, and sudden death.

Short-Term and Long-Term Side Effects/Reasons for Limiting/Quitting

The most common short-term side effects seen with stimulant use occurs when dosages are high (ie, more than 500 mg of caffeine per day) or if several stimulants are used concurrently, or stacked (eg, caffeine, nicotine, and amphetamine). In these situations, athletes may complain of weight loss, headache, irritability, nausea/vomiting, overheating, shakiness, and/or insomnia. These same side effects can be seen when dosages of prescribed medications for ADHD are at the higher end of the dosage range or are used twice daily to try and cover the typical 12 hours to 14 hours in an elite athlete's workday.

The most serious long-term side effects of stimulants include the development of a use disorder (primarily with nicotine, cocaine, and methamphetamine) or paranoia, severe anxiety/panic, psychosis, chronic insomnia, seizure, stroke, or sudden death.

Effects of Performance

The studies that demonstrate a stimulant's performance-enhancing (ergogenic) effects in sports generally are those that use surrogate exercise tasks that have the clearest link to the sports itself (eg, muscle strength for weight lifting and Wingate anaerobic 30-second cycling ergometer test for speed skating). As discussed previously, caffeine improves exercise performance across a broad range of exercise tasks, including muscle endurance, muscle strength, anaerobic power, jumping performance, and exercise speed.[12] Although most studies of caffeine's effects on exercise have been conducted in men, a recent systematic review by Mielgo-Ayuso and colleagues[13] showed that it had similar ergogenic effects on men's and women's aerobic performance and fatigue index but fewer effects in women compared with men on power, total weight lifted, and repeat sprint performance. These effects are thought to be due to caffeine's ability to improve vigilance and alertness, improve neuromuscular function, increase endorphin release, and reduce pain perception and by binding to adenosine receptors in the brain and thereby reducing its fatiguing effects.

Prescribed amphetamine and methylphenidate and supplements containing ephedrine, pseudoephedrine, and phenylpropanolamine improve exercise performance in exercise tasks that are similar to those for caffeine. Studies of prescribed stimulants show positive effects on muscle strength, acceleration, and time to exhaustion in untrained subjects, and positive effects on average power output in time-trial performance in warm weather in trained athletes.

In summary, stimulants may have a positive effect on performance through increased levels of alertness and energy, improved focus and sustained attention, heightened mental quickness, increased stamina, and reduced motor restlessness and emotional impulsivity. This is especially true especially if an athlete had ADH symptoms or disorder or was experiencing jet lag or sleep deprivation.

CANNABIS/CANNABINOIDS

The cannabis plant contains more than 100 natural chemicals called cannabinoids. The 2 major chemicals are delta-9-tetrahydrocannabinol (THC), which is the main psychoactive (high-producing) chemical, and cannabidiol (CBD), which does not produce a high but may have some medicinal properties. There is evidence that cannabis has a variety of therapeutic uses, including the treatment of glaucoma, nausea from chemotherapy, anorexia and wasting (eg. AIDS), chronic pain, inflammation, anxiety, and certain seizure disorders.[14]

CBD is one of many cannabinoids that have been isolated from the marijuana and hemp plants. Hemp-derived CBD is readily available over the counter in all states and can be used via vaping, smoking, oral aerosol, topicals, and tinctures for swallowing. Synthetic cannabinoids are a class of chemicals that bind to the same receptors in the brain as does THC and produce many of the same cannabis-like effects. Their effects usually are much more intense and long-lasting than those of THC and sometimes can be unpredictable. Because of this and their very high potency, even low doses of synthetic cannabinoids can produce toxic effects (eg, paranoia, panic, severe depression, and psychosis). This class of chemicals is extremely dangerous and should be avoided.

The ways to use marijuana have increased over the past 2 decades as the potency has increased. Marijuana can be inhaled as a vapor, smoked, or ingested orally. The typical level of THC in marijuana products are significantly higher now compared with 10 years ago. The THC content for concentrates is the highest, ranging from 50% to 90%. Edibles usually range from 30% to 50% THC content, whereas trimmed flowers are 10% to 25%. The higher the THC level, the greater the likelihood for negative effects.

Prevalence/Reasons for Use

Cannabis containing mainly THC and CBD has become the most widely used illicit substance among athletes, although the rates of use appear to be less than in the general population or similar nonathletic populations.[14,15] One systematic review reported that approximately 23.4% of male athletes and female athletes from different countries in a range of sports (N = 46,202) self-report use in the past year.

Use is more common among male athletes in certain sports (eg, lacrosse, ice hockey, swimming, wrestling, bobsledding, and skeleton) and among those that use it for performance and coping. Not only have the rates of cannabis use in athletes risen over the past decade but also the use of synthetic cannabinoids. In an analysis of 5956 urines from US athletes, Heltsley and colleagues[16] found that 4.5% were positive for the 2 most common synthetic cannabinoids and their metabolites. This is significantly higher than the overall rates of past year use reported in the NCAA study from 2013 (1.6%) and 2017 (0.7%).

The most common self-reported reasons for cannabis use in sports are socialization, stress control, anxiety, depression, anger, relaxation, insomnia, and pain control. The NCAA reports that 77% of student athletes use cannabis for social reasons, 26% as a sleep aid, 22% for anxiety/depression, and 19% for pain management; Zeigler and colleagues[17] study reported similar findings.

Short-Term and Long-Term Side Effects/Reasons for Limiting/Quitting

Despite the view of marijuana as safe or safer than alcohol, approximately 9% of those who use it regularly become addicted.[18] That number almost doubles (17%) among those who start using as teenagers and is 25% to 50% among those who use it daily. Negative effects of short-term use include cough, impaired short-term memory, impaired motor coordination, impaired judgment, and, in high doses, anxiety, panic attacks, paranoia, and psychosis. Negative effects of long-term or heavy use, especially when starting during adolescence, include altered brain development, cognitive impairment, reduced life satisfaction and achievement, and increased risk of a psychotic disorder in persons with a predisposition to such disorders.

Effects on Performance

The literature does not demonstrate an ergogenic effect of cannabis; on the contrary, investigators conclude that cannabis likely diminishes performance by increasing heart rate and blood pressure, decreasing work performance and acutely interfering with steadiness, reaction time, and psychomotor performance. Kennedy[19] conducted a systematic review and identified 15 published studies that showed that THC did not enhance aerobic exercise or strength. Ware and colleagues[20] conducted a nonsystematic review and found that cannabis' effect on performance largely was negative due to its acute negative effects on level of alertness, reaction time, psychomotor agility, and mental quickness (cognition). Its potential to improve sleep, reduce anxiety, reduce inflammation, and manage pain was seen as possibly bene-ficial to performance.

Finally, there appears to be no evidence for performance-enhancing effects from chronic cannabis consumption or cannabidiol use. Kramer and colleagues[21] per-formed a systematic review on chronic cannabis use on physiologic measurements of cardiopulmonary performance in active adults (eg, Vo_{2max} and physical work capac-ity) and found no differences between users and nonusers. McCartney and col-leagues[22] found no studies demonstrating a positive CBD effect on performance or exercise. They concluded that CBD may improve performance indirectly through its anti-inflammatory, neuroprotective, analgesic, and anxiolytic effects, resulting in enhanced healing of traumatic musculoskeletal injuries, improved pain control, reduced anxiety, and improved sleep. WADA has removed CBD from its list of banned substances.

EVOLVING ISSUES IN DOPING IN SPORT AND THE ATHLETE BIOLOGICAL PASSPORT

The ability to manipulate the expression of a functional genes and proteins, along with the ability to influence protein synthesis, is appealing to the performance world. Gene doping is defined as the transfer of cells or genetic elements or the use of pharmaco-logic or biologic agent that alter genes expression. Gene doping has the potential to influence strength, explosiveness, endurance, and recovery. The potential to target specific genes that affect performance or tissue repair is a growing area of interest.

Gene doping may influence muscle fiber type that is associated with strength, po-wer, and explosiveness. IGF-1 and myostatin are genes that appear to influence strength. The ACE gene appears to have associations with cardiac and respiratory function and improve endurance in athletes. EPO and PPAR are specific genes that may affect endurance. An athlete predisposed to an injury may be identified early and gene doping may prevent or minimize an injury with accelerating recovery. This area of science still is developing along with its application.

The ongoing use and evolution of steroids including designer steroids like tetrahy-drogestrinone and SARMs like RAD-140 and ostarine have pushed the antidoping strategies to enhance detection methods. As a result, WADA created the ABP to monitor blood and urine over time with the intent to reveal the effects of doping rather than attempting to detect the doping substance or method itself. The hematological ABP module includes hematocrit, hemoglobin, and several red blood cell indices. The Steroidal Module is used to detect use of AASs. Both modules may detect the in-crease the production of red blood cells that ultimately lead to a performance advan-tage. The steroidal ABP may require isotope ratio mass spectroscopy testing to evaluate the T/E ratio. The Steroidal Module monitors several other metabolites and their levels. The T/E ratio can be influenced by alcohol, 5-alpha reductase inhibitors, aromatase inhibitors, antiestrogens, diuretics, and ketoconazole. The endocrine ABP is in development and targets growth factors, such as IGF-1 and GH. It may prove beneficial in the emerging practice of microdosing when small doses of androgens are used to avoid detection.

MicroRNAs (miRNAs) are small noncoding RNAs that regulate various biological processes. Because circulating miRNAs are highly stable in several body fluids, they hold potential as a new class of biomarkers for the detection of doping and may complement ABP.[23] CRISPR cas9 or similar methods to edit genes may play a pivotal role in doping. To detect gene doping and the consequences of alteration of genetic material, transcriptomics and proteomics may lead the way because they are indicative of gene activity.

In conclusion, sports play an important role in most cultures, and the use of performance-enhancing substance and methods continues to grow. Despite the health risks and the risk of getting caught and paying the consequences, many athletes seek to gain an advantage through doping. The substances are used to enhance mass, endurance, and alertness; accelerate recovery; or manipulate the blood. Other than caffeine, athletes use alcohol more commonly than any other substance. Low doses may assist with performance in some sports, but higher doses usually are detrimental. AASs, SARMs, peptide hormones, growth factors, and metabolic modulators continue to be among the most common findings in an AAF. Stimulants have several performance-enhancing effects. It appears the main reason for opioid use among athletes is to play through pain. Despite the widespread use of cannabis and related products, there are few data to show a benefit on performance however there may be some benefit to reducing pain/inflammation and anxiety and improving sleep.

CLINICS CARE POINTS

- Misuse of any substance class (e.g. alcohol, stimulants, androgens) has characteristic signs and symptoms of use and withdrawal that are keys to detection (see **table 1**).
- Point of care rapid urine tests aid detection for many substance classes and can be done if misuse is suspected.
- Preseason screening for alcohol and other drugs using validated instruments should become routine (e.g. AUDIT-C-alcohol use disorders identification test-consumption questions 1-3, CAGE for drugs).
- Asking open ended questions can facilitate openness (e.g. What is your pattern of using alcohol or other drugs ? What negative consequences from using alcohol or other drugs have you experienced ?).

DISCLOSURE

The authors have no commercial or financial conflicts of interest and any funding sources.

REFERENCES

1. McDuff D, Stull T, Castaldelli-Maia JM, et al. Recreational and ergogenic substance use and substance use disorders in elite athletes: a narrative review. Br J Sports Med 2019;53:754–60.
2. World Anti-Doping Agency. Anti-Doping Testing Figures; 2003-2015, 2017. Available at: https://www.wada-ama.org/en/resources/laboratories/anti-doping-testing-figures-report. Accessed October 16, 2020.
3. Handelsman DJ. Performance Enhancing Hormone Doping in Sport. [Updated 2020 Feb 29]. In: Feingold KR, Anawalt B, Boyce A, et al, editors. Endotext [Internet]. South Dartmouth (MA): MDText.com, Inc.; 2020. Available at: https://www.ncbi.nlm.nih.gov/books/NBK305894/.
4. Fan W, Waizenegger W, Lin CS, et al. PPARδ promotes running endurance by preserving glucose. Cell Metab 2017;25:1186–93.e4.
5. Andrews MA, Magee CD, Combest TM, et al. Physical effects of anabolic-androgenic steroids in healthy exercising adults: a systematic review and meta-analysis. Curr Sports Med Rep 2018;17:232–41.

6. Ford JA, Pomykacz C, Veliz P, et al. Sports involvement, injury history, and non-medical use of prescription opioids among college students: an analysis with a national sample. Am J Addict 2018;27:15–22.

7. Cottler L, Forchheimer R. Injury, pain, and prescription opioid use among former NFL players. Drug Alcohol Dep 2011;116:188–94.

8. Heuberger JAAC, Cohen AF. Review of WADA prohibited substances: limited evidence for performance-enhancing effects. Sports Med 2019;49:525–39.

9. Aguilar-Navarro M, Muñoz G, Salinero JJ, et al. Urine caffeine concentration in doping control samples from 2004 to 2015. Nutrients 2019;11:286.

10. NCAA national Study on Substance Use Habits of Collegiate Student Athletes. 2018. Available at: http://www.ncaa.org/sites/default/files/2018RES_Substance_Use_Final_Report_FINAL_20180611.pdf. Accessed October 8, 2020.

11. Martin T. Report of major league baseball's joint drug prevention and treatment program. 2018. Available at: http://www.mlb.com/documents/3/8/2/301315382/IPA_2018_Public_Report_113018.pdf. Accessed October 8, 2020.

12. Baltazar-Martins JG, Brito de Souza D, Aguilar M, et al. Infographic. The road to the ergogenic effect of caffeine on exercise performance. Br J Sports Med 2020; 54:618–9.

13. Mielgo-Ayuso J, Marques-Jiménez D, Refoyo I, et al. Effect of caffeine supplementation on sports performance based on differences between sexes: a systematic review. Nutrients 2019;11:2313.

14. Docter S, Khan M, Gohal C, et al. Cannabis use and sport: a systematic review. Sports Health 2020;12:189–99.

15. Brisola-Santos MB, de Mello e Gallinaro JG, Gil F, et al. Prevalence and correlates of cannabis use among athletes-A systematic review. Am J Addict 2016;25:518–28.

16. Heltsley R, Shelby MK, Crouch DJ, et al. Prevalence of synthetic cannabinoids in U.S. athletes: initial findings. J Anal Toxicol 2012;36:588–93.

17. Zeigler J, Silvers W, Fleegler E, Zeigler R. Age related differences in cannabis use and subjective effects in a large population-based survey of adult athletes. J Cannabis Res 2019;1:7.

18. Volkow ND, Baler RD, Compton WM, et al. Adverse health effects of marijuana use. N Engl J Med 2014;370:2219–37.

19. Kennedy MC. Cannabis: exercise performance and sport. a systematic review. J Sci Med Sport 2017;20(9):825–9.

20. Ware MA, Jensen D, Barrette A, et al. Cannabis and the Health and Performance of the Elite Athlete. Clin J Sport Med 2018;28(5):480–4.

21. Kramer A, Sinclair J, Sharpe L, et al. Chronic cannabis consumption and physical exercise performance in healthy adults: a systematic review. J Cannabis Res 2020;2(34):1–8.

22. McCartney D, Benson MJ, Desbrow B, et al. Cannabidiol and Sports Performance: a Narrative Review of Relevant Evidence and Recommendations for Future Research. Sports Med Open 2020;6:27.

23. Leuenberger N, Robinson N, Saugy M. Circulating miRNAs: a new generation of anti-doping biomarkers. Anal Bioanal Chem 2013;405:9617–23.

Attention-Deficit/ Hyperactivity Disorder and Sports: A Lifespan Perspective

Lisa MacLean, MD[a], Deepak Prabhakar, MD, MPH[b],*

KEYWORDS

- ADHD • Athletes • Life span • Sport Psychiatry

KEY POINTS

- There is no standardized objective measure to make the diagnosis of attention-deficit/ hyperactivity disorder (ADHD); the diagnosis is made with a thorough clinical history.
- Patients suffering from ADHD have twice the lifetime risk of substance use disorders compared with their non-ADHD peers.
- For athletes, the type of sport, level of play, and baseline health should be considered in the decision to use medications for the treatment of ADHD.
- The use of stimulants, although beneficial in athletes, is not without risk and potential for cardiovascular and thermoregulatory adverse events.
- In professional athletes who need treatment of ADHD, nonstimulants should be carefully considered; when stimulants are used, long-acting stimulants are preferred.

INTRODUCTION

Attention-deficit/hyperactivity disorder (ADHD) is a chronic and pervasive heritable neurobiological developmental disorder that can affect an individual throughout their life span. For diagnosis, the core symptoms of ADHD are hyperactivity, impulsivity, and/or inattention that emerge by age 12 years, cannot be due to another mental or medical condition, and cause impairment in at least 2 settings. ADHD affects about 5% of the general population younger than 19 years and about 4% of adults.[1] Because of its prevalence and negative impact on multiple domains over the course of a person's life, ADHD is considered a major health problem. The chapter provides an overview of ADHD from preschool to the adult years with a focus on its impact on athletes. It will also provide context to the progressive and changing needs of the patient with treatment recommendations for an athlete throughout every stage of their athletic career.

[a] Henry Ford Health System, One Ford Place, 1C, Detroit, MI 48202, USA; [b] Sheppard Pratt, 6501 North Charles Street, Baltimore, MD 21204, USA
* Corresponding author.
E-mail address: dprabhakar@sheppardpratt.org

Psychiatr Clin N Am 44 (2021) 419–430
https://doi.org/10.1016/j.psc.2021.04.014
0193-953X/21/© 2021 Elsevier Inc. All rights reserved.

ATTENTION-DEFICIT/HYPERACTIVITY DISORDER ACROSS THE LIFE SPAN

ADHD occurs in approximately 2% to 5% of children in the preschool age group.[2] The impairments seen at this age are similar to those seen in older school age children.[3] ADHD in these age groups is characterized by inattentive, hyperactive, and impulsive behaviors. Struggling with social relationships and learning are common impairments seen in these children; they commonly interrupt conversations, have poor coordination, and blurt out inappropriate comments. They are also more likely to be suspended, be in accidents, and sustain injuries.[4] Preschoolers and older school age children also demonstrate similar levels of psychiatric comorbidities, with the most common being learning and language disabilities, oppositional defiant disorder, conduct disorder, depression, and anxiety disorders.[5] These behaviors can result in poor peer relationships, which can lead to further isolation and low self-esteem affecting the child academically and within the family unit. Research suggests that the younger the age of onset of symptoms, the more likely the disorder will be severe during childhood.[6] Children who receive treatment have a better prognosis than those who do not.[7]

Approximately 50% of children will continue to meet diagnostic criteria for ADHD into adolescence. However, with development, hyperactivity, although still present, lessens in severity. Developmentally, adolescence is a time when decisions about life choices are made that could both positively and negatively affect an individual's future. In high school, adolescents must learn to function in an environment that is often more demanding and less structured. The influence of peers becomes particularly important and issues around poor self-regulation can create difficulty. In addition, several comorbid problems may arise that require treatment, such as antisocial personality characteristics, depression, anxiety, and substance abuse problems.[8] In an empirically based literature review, Gillberg and colleagues found that beginning in their adolescent years, patients suffering from ADHD have twice the lifetime risk of substance abuse compared with their non-ADHD peers.[9] The adolescent years are a time of transition when a young person learns of their personal responsibility for their actions. By age 21 years, 95% of teenagers stop taking medication, and this decline is unlikely due to resolution of symptoms,[10] and this puts adolescent patients with ADHD at greater risk for negative outcomes and could slow the successful transition from adolescence to adulthood.

The estimated point prevalence of ADHD is about 4% in the adult general population.[11] Thus, a substantial proportion of young adults continue to have symptoms or associated problems that may require treatment. Indeed, current estimates suggest that about half of the patients with childhood ADHD continue with symptoms into adulthood.[11] Similar to adolescence, impulsivity and hyperactivity tend to abate, but attentional problems persist into adulthood.[12] Adults often experience more difficulty with procrastination, time management, and organization, which can be particularly problematic for college students. Furthermore, most adults with ADHD can experience multiple negative life events related to academic underachievement, problematic driving, underemployment or recurrent unemployment, imprisonment, and problems with forming and maintaining relationships.[13] Comorbid problems include mood and anxiety disorders, emotional dysregulation, low frustration tolerance, irritability, anger, insomnia, increased risk taking, and problems with alcohol and substance misuse. Impulsivity may place patients at greater risk to injure themselves, resulting in higher rates of traumatic brain injury and other injuries (**Table 1**).

ADHD symptoms often start in the preschool years, but children tend to be diagnosed only after entering school, when the difficulties of meeting the academic demands become apparent and the child exhibits behavioral or cognitive deficits. The male-female prevalence ratio of the disorder is 3:1 in children with equal male-to-female ratios in adults.[11] Because there is no standardized objective measure to make the diagnosis of ADHD, the diagnosis is made after a thorough clinical history. Review of standardized validated symptomatology questionnaires can help the diagnostic evaluation.

Patient evaluation regardless of the age should include gathering collateral information from parents, teachers, and in adults, partners or coworkers. When making the diagnosis, it is also important to screen for psychiatric and cardiac and other medical comorbidities to ensure that medications, if indicated, can be safely prescribed. The clinician should assess and compare the person's behavior with developmental norms in multiple settings including home, work, and school to ensure that function and impairment warrant intervention. Following the clinical diagnosis, the individual can be assigned a treatment that is tailored to their needs.

ATTENTION-DEFICIT/HYPERACTIVITY DISORDER ACROSS THE LIFE SPAN OF AN ATHLETE
Preschool and Elementary Years

ADHD is a common psychiatric disorder in both the general population and in athletes. Young athletes are a unique patient population. The preschool and elementary years

Table 1
Attention-deficit/hyperactivity disorder concerns over a life span

Age of Patient	Developmental Impact
Preschool	• Behavioral disturbance
School-age	• Behavioral disturbance • Poor social interactions • Academic difficulty • Poor peer acceptance • Comorbid conditions
Adolescent	• Low self-esteem • Poor social interactions • Impulsivity • Academic difficulty • Smoking/substance use • Comorbid conditions
College-age	• Low self-esteem • Academic difficulty • Substance abuse • Injury/accidents • Relationship problems
Adult	• Low self-esteem • Not coping with tasks such as bill paying • Unemployment or underemployment • Relationship problems • Driving issues • Substance abuse • Mood instability • Imprisonment

are the most likely time for the diagnosis of ADHD. Young athletes may experience more problems with balance and coordinated activity.[14] These children often present with behavior issues, which contribute to strain on the parent, child, and family; this strain may result in the subsequent development of depression, self-blame, and social isolation in the parent.

Hyperactivity is more common in children than in adults. In one quasi-experimental study comparing 34 male children (6–17 years) with ADHD with 41 children without ADHD, Johnson and Rosen found that male athletes with ADHD displayed higher levels of aggression, emotional reactivity, and frequency of disqualification.[15] In one retrospective review, children with ADHD were also more likely to be injured than children without ADHD in noncompetitive play.[16] Nevertheless, sports can be a good outlet for children with excess energy, and many kids find that playing sports is a place where they can excel. In addition, research has shown that exercise may decrease inattention and impulsive behaviors.[17] Organized sports can be helpful in providing structure, expectations, and rules. Participation in sports has also been shown to decrease symptoms of anxiety and depression.[18] The impact of a positive coaching experience is one way to build on the confidence of those struggling with ADHD who may have low self-esteem.

Middle School and High School Years

As athletes develop and enter adolescence, the unique challenges of this age group could emerge especially for those with ADHD. For middle school and high school athletes, with parental consent, the coaching staff should be informed about the diagnosis of ADHD and whether the athlete is taking medication. This important information allows the staff to monitor the athlete during practice and competition for potential negative side effects. The designated sport and position need to be considered in the overall treatment decisions for an athlete with ADHD. At this level of play, participation is more important than competition. Being part of a team, learning new skills, and enjoying physical activity typically outweigh the value of winning. This, in combination with academic requirements and success, needs to be considered when creating a comprehensive treatment plan.

College Athletes

Although symptoms of ADHD may be present before college, some students do not receive a diagnosis of ADHD until they are challenged by the academic expectations of the college environment. Greater independence, more temptations for unhealthy behaviors, a lack of parental regulation, lack of structure, and the need for more personal time management could lead to the surfacing of issues related to undiagnosed ADHD, all compounding the athlete's ability to succeed. Because by this age many people experience an abatement of the hyperactivity symptoms, the predominant presentation includes low attention, focus, and concentration. Previous school records, reports from people who know the athlete, and current stressors can all aid in making the diagnosis.

Professional Athletes

The prevalence of ADHD in elite athletes is challenging to determine because the stigma against mental health assessment and treatment is strong within this population.[19] Unfortunately, poor focus, low frustration tolerance, low self-esteem, argumentativeness, and mood lability found in ADHD could impair the performance of an elite athlete, making the diagnosis and treatment of this disorder critical to their success. A review by Regnart and colleagues showed that mood disorders and substance use disorders are also common in adult athletes with ADHD.[20] Screening for these conditions is an important part of the elite athlete's health management strategy.

ATTENTION-DEFICIT/HYPERACTIVITY DISORDER TREATMENT OPTIONS

The ADHD literature describes a wide variety of psychological treatments, with or without the use of stimulant and nonstimulant medication options. Psychological treatment interventions include supportive psychotherapy, cognitive behavior therapy, support groups, parent training, educator/teacher training, biofeedback, medications, and social skills training. The National Institute of Mental Health Multimodal Treatment of ADHD study showed that the use of stimulants was more efficacious than psychosocial management alone, combined treatment, and routine care in the community.[21] Approximately 75% of those with ADHD note some benefit with psychostimulants,[22] and thus, if diagnosed correctly, treatment of ADHD with a stimulant is a favored approach.

Stimulants act on the neurotransmitters that block the reuptake of dopamine and norepinephrine that are responsible for increasing attention and concentration. Stimulants also have a rapid onset, typically within 1 hour, with various durations of action depending on the formulation, giving patients an almost immediate effect. There is also some role for nonstimulant medications such as atomoxetine, bupropion, and guanfacine for patients in whom stimulants may not be an option (**Table 2**). The major benefit to nonstimulants is the absence of both psychological and physiologic abuse concerns. However, in clinical practice, many patients report that nonstimulant options are not as effective at reducing their symptoms as stimulants.

The age of the patient can affect the treatment recommendation. According to a review by Young and Amarasinghe, the most appropriate treatment of preschoolers is parent training.[23] For school-aged children with moderate impairment, group parent training and classroom behavioral interventions are typically recommended. For more severe impairment, these interventions are more appropriate when combined with stimulant medication. In considering the development of a comprehensive treatment plan, behavioral treatment can be particularly effective. Behavioral treatments for younger children should include consequences that are concrete, frequent, and coincide directly with the concerning behavior, and this allows the child to connect their negative behavior with the consequence. For older children, cognitive skills training can be taught to address social and achievement-related issues and will give the child some autonomy and ownership in their treatment.

Interventions that include the integration of home and school strategies, psychopharmacology, and some component of social skills training are best suited for middle school and adolescent children. For adolescence, treatment decisions cannot simply be imposed by an authority figure. Accepting medication needs to be negotiated and agreed on by the adolescent whose collaboration and agreement is critical to ensure treatment compliance.

Stimulant medication is generally first-line treatment of adults, but cognitive behavioral therapy coaching, group therapy, and marital therapy have also been found to be helpful. Regardless of the developmental stage, for patients to experience the highest level of remission and symptom abatement, treatments must also address the individual's daily adaptive functioning and their comorbid problems.

As individuals move into late adolescence and adulthood, treatments involving a cognitive behavioral perspective are likely to become increasingly helpful.[23] Recommendations regarding academic support and accommodations should be considered a necessary part of the treatment plan. Regardless of the age of the individual,

Table 2
Common attention-deficit/hyperactivity disorder medications and common side effects

Category	Generic Name	Trade Name	Common Side Effects
Stimulants	Methylphenidate	Concerta, Ritalin, Metadata, Focalin, Methylin, Quillivant, Daytrana	Decreased appetite, weight loss, sleep difficulties, nervousness, irritability, hypertension, tachycardia
	Mixed dextroamphetamine-amphetamine salts	Adderall, Adderall XR, Mydayis	Decreased appetite, weight loss, sleep difficulties, nervousness, irritability, hypertension, tachycardia
	Dextroamphetamine	Dexedrine, Dextrostat	Decreased appetite, weight loss, sleep difficulties, nervousness, irritability, hypertension, tachycardia
	Lisdextroamphetamine	Vyvanse	Decreased appetite, weight loss, sleep difficulties, nervousness, irritability, hypertension, tachycardia
Nonstimulants	Atomoxetine HCL	Strattera	Fatigue, sedation, dry mouth, GI upset, increased sweating, hypertension. Rarely increased suicidality and hepatotoxic
	Bupropion	Wellbutrin, Zyban	Anorexia, tics, nervousness, potential seizures
	Guanfacine	Intuniv, Tenex	Sleepiness, drowsiness, dizziness, headache, irritability, low blood pressure, nausea, stomach pain, dry mouth, constipation, and decreased appetite

Abbreviation: GI, gastrointestinal.

clinicians should ensure that the goals and method of treatment are tangible and motivating. Thus, treatments should be modified at key developmental transitions using developmentally sensitive strategies that place the patient's most debilitating behaviors in the context of their level of understanding and ability to participate in their treatment.

COMMON MEDICATION SIDE EFFECTS

The benefit of stimulants must be weighed against the potential risks. Common side effects include decreased appetite, headache, gastrointestinal upset, and insomnia.

Cardiovascular side effects include rapid heart rate and increased blood pressure. There has been concern of sudden cardiac death from the use of stimulants for ADHD. However, review of the literature by Perrin and colleagues did not support this, and in 2008, a policy statement in the American Academy of Pediatrics recommended electrocardiogram screening only if there are concerning history or physical examination findings or a strong family history of predisposing cardiac conditions.[24] Prescribing clinicians should take a careful personal and family cardiac history and monitor the athlete's blood pressure and heart rate both before initiating treatment and during follow-up appointments (**Box 1**).

Another potential side effect of stimulants is the increased risk of heat illness, which is a common cause of death in athletes.[25] It is associated with physical activity and defined as the body's inability to regulate and offset the increase in core body temperature. The risk of developing heat illness increases for athletes on stimulants because of their effects on the body's regulatory system, interfering with normal thermoregulation by altering neurotransmitter activity in the brain. When prescribing stimulants to athletes, clinicians should monitor the athlete's weight and vital signs, alert them of the risk of heat illness, and educate them on the signs of heat-related illness, especially for those who participate in activities requiring sustained cardiovascular exertion such as cycling or cross-country running.

ATTENTION-DEFICIT/HYPERACTIVITY DISORDER AND CONCUSSION

There is an overlap in the clinical presentations of ADHD and concussion. In a cross-sectional study of 8056 high school and collegiate athletes, Nelson found that individuals with ADHD had a greater rate of baseline fatigue, poor concentration, insomnia, difficulty remembering, and balance problems, all of which can mimic the symptoms of a concussion.[26] This study also found that ADHD and learning disabilities place an athlete at 2 to 3 times the risk for repetitive concussive injuries. In addition, individuals with ADHD have been reported to have a continued decline on repeat neurocognitive testing scores after concussion.[27] A study by Biederman comparing 29 student athletes with ADHD with a historical sample of subjects without ADHD suggested that

---

Box 1
Cardiovascular screening

Personal History Questions
1. What is your history of heart murmurs, hypertension, chest pain, and palpitations?
2. Do you have a history of structural cardiac defects?
3. Have you ever had a cardiac event?
4. When was your last EKG? What were the results?
5. Have you ever had a history of any cardiac disease?
6. Have you ever had a history of any respiratory disease?

Family History Questions
1. Is there any family history of cardiac disease?
2. Has anyone in your family ever died young of a cardiac disease?

Cardiovascular Examination
1. Measure heart rate
2. Measure blood pressure
3. Cardiac auscultation looking for murmur
4. EKG if any of the aforementioned history is positive

Abbreviation: EKG, electrocardiogram.

this may be due to worsening inattention from ADHD rather than from concussion although this is a complex analysis, as concussion itself can cause inattention.[28] Furthermore, ADHD has been reported to slow the recovery of a concussion for up to 3 days.[29] Although recovery can be lengthened, some research shows that there does not seem to be a risk of developing chronic or worsened ADHD symptoms after concussion, whereas other research showed that children with ADHD had more significant symptoms of inattention after a closed head injury than controls.[25]

All of these points make the evaluation and management of concussion more complex in this patient population. The prolonged recovery time and confusing clinical picture can make it difficult to determine when it is safe to recommend the athlete return to academics and to play. Therefore, clinicians should proceed with caution and consider a multidisciplinary approach. If at the time of injury, symptoms are well controlled, despite limited evidence, accepted practice is to continue medications.[30]

SPECIAL TREATMENT CONSIDERATIONS FOR ATHLETES

When prescribing treatment of athletes, there are unique challenges that must be considered. The clinician caring for these athletes must customize care and treatment recommendations to accommodate an athlete's needs. Because the presentation, diagnosis, and treatment of athletes can change across the life span, the age of the athlete, their health status, student status, and the severity of their symptoms must be taken into consideration by the treating clinician. Except in very young athletes, stimulant medication with or without a psychological intervention is generally first-line treatment of ADHD. Because of high levels of intense exercise and activity, the physiologic and potential psychological effects of stimulants on athletes is a valid concern. When considering a stimulant medication, risk of diversion and potential for abuse should also be considered. For these reasons, long-acting agents should be considered as first-line stimulant treatment.

In children and adolescents, coaching that is structured and organized will result in the greatest benefit. Complicated instructions may need to be broken down into smaller pieces. Rules may need to be repeated. The home environment can play a major role, and homes that provide structure, calmness, and consistency can help a child or adolescent with ADHD perform their best.

Athletics and academics present an interesting dynamic; athletes with ADHD may be more attracted to physical activity than to academics because of inherent restlessness, internal reward-seeking benefits, and natural drive for competitiveness. Conversely, the struggle in the academic setting can lead to low confidence and poor self-esteem. It cannot be overstated that effective treatment not only improves quality of life and academic performance but also has demonstrated a decrease in the rate of substance abuse, driving errors, and the prevalence of comorbid psychological disorders. Balancing the dilemma between patient needs and the potential for serious side effects and unfair advantage in play due to stimulant use should be considered when deciding whether to recommend a stimulant or other nonstimulant strategies and psychological interventions.

In terms of the treatment of ADHD in college-aged or professional athletes, many sports leagues and organizations follow the guidelines established by the World Anti-Doping Agency, which allows therapeutic use exemption (TUE) to permit athletes to take stimulants if deemed necessary by their physicians.[31] TUE is a newer policy, as stimulants were previously listed on the World Anti-Doping Agency–banned list due to their ergogenic potential. For athletes participating in college sports under the supervision of the National College Athletic Association (NCCA), stimulants require TUE in order for athletes to take stimulants without sanction.[32] There has been much controversy and confusion about the rules and regulations around the use of stimulants by these governing bodies. Although the nonstimulant option, atomoxetine, is US Food and Drug Administration approved for the treatment of ADHD, neither governing body requires a trial of atomoxetine before a stimulant trial.[33]

Rates of use of stimulants by NCAA college athletes is not inconsequential. A drug use survey done in 2012 by the NCAA indicated that 4.3% of student athletes reported using stimulants with a prescription, whereas 6.3% of student athletes reported using stimulants without a physician's prescription, leaving the possibility that medication may be given to or sold to the athlete by friends and peers.[34] Abuse of stimulants for recreation and performance improvement is a valid concern.

Treatment decisions in the elite athlete are complicated by concerns related to fair competition. At this level of competition even the tiniest advantage can make a significant difference between winning or losing. When prescribing stimulants in professional sports, clinicians must follow the specific guidelines for therapeutic use exemptions outlined by professional organizations such as Major League Baseball and the National Football League.[35,36] However, a bigger question is whether performance-enhancing agents should even be allowed at the elite level of sports. With the goal of fair play central to any sport, Reardon and Factor argue that all performance-enhancing agents including stimulants should either be completely prohibited or only prohibited during practice and play, thereby removing some of the ethical and medical concerns associated with their use.[33] Garner and colleagues argue that the banning of stimulants does not necessarily guarantee fair play and may contribute to poor social functioning and low self-esteem.[37] When making this decision, one should consider the evidence for increased risk of injury during play in inattentive athletes who are not being treated with effective medications.

The severity of symptoms and degree of impairment need to be considered when deciding whether to prescribe stimulants in a professional athlete. If medication is clinically necessary for an elite athlete, nonstimulant medication, such as atomoxetine, should be explored. For athletes with comorbid depression, there is some clinical evidence that bupropion, an antidepressant with some stimulant properties, may be helpful as an off-label for the treatment of ADHD.

Regardless of the age of the ADHD athlete, the designated sport and position need to be considered in the overall treatment decisions. Working with the athlete on the timing of the medication, such that it is most effective during academic sessions, should be explored. As a clinician, when providing treatment, the main goal is to develop a strategy that helps the athlete achieve success both academically and as an athlete, while remaining compliant with published sports governing body regulations. This customized strategy makes sense when the athlete is also a student and must obtain continued academic success in order to advance. However, when the athlete is an adult playing a professional sport, the use of stimulants should be used only after careful consideration. In making this decision, clinicians should consider issues related to the likelihood of performance enhancement, accuracy of the ADHD diagnosis, policies of sports governing bodies and potential for diversion and abuse.

SUMMARY

ADHD is a common neurodevelopmental psychiatric disorder that affects both athletes and nonathletes. Those with ADHD who participate in sports find that it can be mutually beneficial, as these individuals can naturally excel as well as have an outlet for symptom management. The diagnosis and treatment of ADHD is critical to the optimal functioning and quality of life of those who struggle with this condition. The focus of treatment should be on psychological interventions with or without medications. The use of stimulants should be carefully reviewed and factor in the age, level of play and sport, and the health of the athlete. If stimulants are used, long-acting stimulants are preferred as first-line stimulant treatment.

Psychological interventions such as cognitive behavioral therapy, individual education plans; behavior modification therapy; caregiver support; parent teaching/training; and ADHD education for the patient, family, and coaches should be explored and recommended. In addition to these interventions, a comprehensive treatment plan should also include recommendations for healthy nutrition and physical exercise, as data have supported the benefit of both of these strategies. When impairment is moderate or severe, psychostimulant medication still remains first-line treatment of the abatement of ADHD symptoms. Treatment should not be avoided in student athletes. In professional athletes, treatment with stimulants should only be used after carefully weighing the risks and benefits, and nonstimulants should be carefully considered. Ultimately, pharmacotherapy with or without psychosocial interventions play a fundamental role in the management of ADHD athletes across their life span.

CLINICS CARE POINTS

- Younger children and athletes with ADHD, often present with comorbid behavioral problems.
- Unmitigated ADHD impacts performance in sports and academic/ vocational tasks.
- Age-appropriate psychosocial interventions should be considered along with medication management.
- Healthy nutrition, sleep hygiene and physical exercise related education should be included in a treatment plan for ADHD.
- Stimulant medications are highly effective and should be considered in athletes after judicious review of clinical presentation.
- Practitioners treating collegiate, amateur and professional athletes should make themselves aware of specific regulations of the specific sport governing bodies.

DISCLOSURE

The authors have nothing to disclose.

REFERENCES

1. Polanczyk G, de Lima MS, Horta BL, et al. The worldwide prevalence of ADHD: a systematic review and metaregression analysis. Am J Psychiatry 2007;164: 942–8.
2. Lavigne JV, Gibbons RD, Christoffel KK, et al. Prevalence rates and correlates of psychiatric disorders among preschool children. J Am Acad Child Adolesc Psychiatry 1996;35:204–14.
3. Sonuga-Barke EJ, Dalen L, Remington B. Do executive deficits and delay aversion make independent contributions to preschool attention-deficit/hyperactivity disorder symptoms? J Am Acad Child Adolesc Psychiatry 2003;42:1335–42.
4. Egger HL, Kondo D, Angold A. The epidemiology and diagnostic issues in preschool attention-deficit/hyperactivity disorder: a review. Infants Young Child 2006;19:109–22.

5. Ford T, Goodman R, Meltzer H. The british child and adolescent mental health survey 1999: the prevalence of DSM-IV disorders. J Am Acad Child Adolesc Psychiatry 2003;42:1203–11.

6. Sonuga-Barke EJS, Thompson M, Abikoff H, et al. Nonpharmacological interventions for preschoolers with ADHD. Infants Young Child 2006;19:142–53.

7. Lahey BB, Pelham WE, Stein MA, et al. Validity of DSM-IV attention-deficit/hyperactivity disorder for younger children. J Am Acad Child Adolesc Psychiatry 1998; 37:695–702.

8. Fischer M, Barkley RA, Smallish L, et al. Young adult follow-up of hyperactive children: self-reported psychiatric disorders, comorbidity, and the role of childhood conduct problems and teen CD. J Abnorm Child Psychol 2002;30:463–75.

9. Gillberg C, Gillberg IC, Rasmussen P, et al. Co-existing disorders in ADHD – implications for diagnosis and intervention. Eur Child Adolesc Psychiatry 2004; 13(Suppl 1):l80–92.

10. McCarthy S, Asherson P, Coghill D, et al. Attention-deficit hyperactivity disorder: treatment discontinuation in adolescents and young adults. Br J Psychiatry 2009; 194:273–7.

11. Kessler RC, Adler L, Barkley R, et al. The prevalence and correlates of adult ADHD in the United States: results from the National Comorbidity Survey Replication. Am J Psychiatry 2006;163:716–23.

12. Biederman J, Mick E, Faraone SV. Age-dependent decline of symptoms of attention deficit hyperactivity disorder: impact of remission definition and symptom type. Am J Psychiatry 2000;157:816–8.

13. Wilens TE, Faraone SV, Biederman J. Attention-deficit/hyperactivity disorder in adults. JAMA 2004;292:619–23.

14. Archer T, Kostrzewa RM. Physical exercise alleviates ADHD symptoms: regional deficits and development trajectory. Neurotox Res 2012;21:195–209.

15. Johnson RC, Rosen LA. Sports behavior of ADHD children. J Atten Disord 2000; 4:150–60.

16. DiScala C, Lescohier I, Barthel M, et al. Injuries to children with attention deficit hyperactivity disorder. Pediatrics 1998;102:1415–21.

17. Halperin JM, Healey DM. The influences of environmental enrichment, cognitive enhancement, and physical exercise on brain development: can we alter the developmental trajectory of ADHD? Neurosci Biobehav Rev 2011;35:621–34.

18. Kiluk BD, Weden S, Culotta VP. Sport participation and anxiety in children with ADHD. J Atten Disord 2009;12:499–506.

19. Putukian M, Kreher JB, Coppel DB, et al. Attention deficit hyperactivity disorder and the athlete: an American Medical Society for Sports Medicine position statement. Clin J Sport Med 2011;21:392–401.

20. Regnart J, Truter I, Meyer A. Critical exploration of co-occurring attention-deficit/hyperactivity disorder, mood disorder and substance use disorder. Expert Rev Pharmacoecon Outcomes Res 2017;17:275–82.

21. National Institute of Mental Health Multimodal Treatment Study of ADHD followup: 24-month outcomes of treatment strategies for attention-deficit/hyperactivity disorder; MTA Cooperative Group. Pediatrics 2004;113(4):754–61.

22. Sallee FR, Gill HS. Neuropsychopharmacology III: psychostimulants. In: Coffey CE, Brumback RA, editors. Textbook of pediatric neuropsychiatry. Washington, DC: American Psychiatry Press; 1998. p. 1351–72.

23. Young S, Amarasinghe JM. Practitioner review: Non-pharmacological treatments for ADHD: a lifespan approach. J Child Psychol Psychiatry 2010;51:116–33.

24. Perrin JM, Friedman RA, Knilans TK, Black Box Working G, Section on C, Cardiac S. Cardiovascular monitoring and stimulant drugs for attention-deficit/hyperactivity disorder. Pediatrics 2008;122:451–3.

25. Stewman CG, Liebman C, Fink L, et al. Attention deficit hyperactivity disorder: unique considerations in athletes. Sports Health 2018;10:40–6.

26. Nelson LD, Guskiewicz KM, Marshall SW, et al. Multiple self-reported concussions are more prevalent in athletes with ADHD and learning disability. Clin J Sport Med 2016;26:120–7.

27. Cottle JE, Hall EE, Patel K, et al. Concussion baseline testing: preexisting factors, symptoms, and neurocognitive performance. J Athl Train 2017;52:77–81.

28. Biederman J, Feinberg L, Chan J, et al. Mild traumatic brain injury and attention-deficit hyperactivity disorder in young student athletes. J Nerv Ment Dis 2015; 203:813–9.

29. Levin H, Hanten G, Max J, et al. Symptoms of attention-deficit/hyperactivity disorder following traumatic brain injury in children. J Dev Behav Pediatr 2007;28: 108–18.

30. Harmon KG, Drezner JA, Gammons M, et al. American Medical Society for Sports Medicine position statement: concussion in sport. Br J Sports Med 2013;47: 15–26.

31. World Anti-Doping Agency. Medical Information to support the decisions of TUE Committees attention deficit hyperactivity disorder (ADHD) in children and adults (Version 5.0). Available at: https://www.wada-ama.org/sites/default/files/resources/files/WADA-MI-ADHD-5.0.pdf. Accessed October 2, 2020.

32. Parr JW. Attention-deficit hyperactivity disorder and the athlete: new advances and understanding. Clin Sports Med 2011;30:591–610.

33. Reardon CL, Factor RM. Considerations in the use of stimulants in sport. Sports Med 2016;46:611–7.

34. Hendrickson B. Non-medical use of ADHD meds examined in Convention session. Available at: http://www.ncaa.org/about/resources/media-center/news/non-medical-use-adhd-meds-examined-convention-session. Accessed October 2, 2020.

35. Major League Baseball. Major League Baseball's joint drug prevention and treatment program. Accessed October 1, 2020. Available at: http://www.mlb.com/pa/pdf/jda.pdf.

36. National Football League. Policy on performance-enhancing substances. Available at: https://nflpaweb.blob.core.windows.net/media/Default/PDFs/Agents/2016PESPolicy_v2.PDF. Accessed October 1, 2020.

37. Garner AA, Hansen AA, Baxley C, et al. The use of stimulant medication to treat attention-deficit/hyperactivity disorder in elite athletes: a performance and health perspective. Sports Med 2018;48:507–12.

Nutrition, Eating Disorders, and Behavior in Athletes

Adena Neglia, MS, RDN, CDN[a,b,*]

KEYWORDS

- Relative energy deficiency in sport (RED-S) • Disordered eating
- Low energy availability • Eating disorders • Body image • Family-based therapy

KEY POINTS

- Sports dietitians play an important role in translating the latest nutrition information for athletes, coaches, and other members of the performance team.
- Eating disorders do not discriminate and can occur in any gender, any sport, any race, any ethnicity, any socioeconomic status, and at any weight or body size.
- Eating disorders are extremely complex and dangerous mental health illnesses and require a specialized treatment team.
- A lower weight or body fat percentage does not always lead to enhanced performance. It can often negatively affect strength, energy levels, focus, and exercise recovery.

INTRODUCTION

More now than ever, athletes are understanding the important role that nutrition has in performance. There are more sports drinks, bars, gels, and supplements than ever before, and anything an athlete wants to research about nutrition, can be found in less than 20 seconds on a smart phone or a computer. With so much information at their fingertips and new diet trends every year, it can be difficult for athletes to determine how best to manage their diets to maximize performance. Without proper guidance or education, a new eating plan may negatively affect performance and recovery, especially if a food group is limited or taken out, or if overall calorie intake is inadequate.

One thing athletes often forget is that their dietary needs are much higher than those of the general population. Individual dietary requirements vary depending on the type of sport, the athlete's goals, body composition, training schedule, environment, and metabolism. Although it is easy to find a calorie calculator or meal plan online, those tools often do not take into consideration all of the mentioned variables, nor do they always take into consideration the athlete's dietary preferences or lifestyle outside

^a Brown & Medina Nutrition, New York, NY, USA; ^b Performance 360, Mount Sinai, NY, USA
* Performance 360, Mount Sinai, NY.
E-mail address: adena@nutritionbyadena.com

Psychiatr Clin N Am 44 (2021) 431–441
https://doi.org/10.1016/j.psc.2021.04.009
0193-953X/21/© 2021 Elsevier Inc. All rights reserved.

psych.theclinics.com

of sports, and this is where working with a sports dietitian can be key. Getting professional help can save both time and money in the long run and prevent athletes from using the wrong (or even harmful) information.

The role of the sports dietitian is to translate the best available evidence into practical nutrition recommendations for the athlete. Sports dietitians can provide individualized nutrition plans, educate athletes on proper supplement use, dispel the latest nutrition myths, and serve as a resource for coaches, trainers, and other team members. They may also coordinate with the team chef to create high-performance menus, choose snacks and beverages for the training room and/or meal room, and even work with hotel staff to create menus while the team is on the road. Although not all sports dietitians receive in-depth training for eating disorders, they play an important role in identifying red flags that come up with regard to athletes' relationships to food and their bodies. This article discusses the fundamentals of nutrition and how nutritionists and the Sport Psychiatrists/Psychologists can work as a team in maximizing mind-body performance.

PATHOPHYSIOLOGY

Although there are always new diets and nutrition trends emerging every year, the basic recommendations for sports nutrition have largely stayed the same over the last few decades. As mentioned earlier, different athletes have different physical demands and nutritional requirements, so customization is key.

The Role of Carbohydrates

Whether an athlete plays ice hockey, football, basketball, or any other high-intensity sport, carbohydrates are going to be the main source of energy, or fuel. During digestion, carbohydrates are broken down into glucose, a simple sugar. Glucose circulates in the blood stream, providing energy to the brain and the nervous system. Glucose can also be converted to glycogen, a stored form of carbohydrate found mostly in the liver and muscles. During heavy exercise, muscle stores of glycogen can easily be depleted, leaving athletes feeling fatigued, weak, and unable to perform at their best.

Carbohydrates should be on every athlete's plate before, after, and at times, during exercise. The preexercise meal should contain 1 to 4 g of carbohydrate per kilogram of body weight and be consumed 1 to 4 hours before training. To prevent any gastrointestinal discomfort while training, it is best to aim for smaller amounts the closer the athlete gets to exercise. Athletes should be careful to limit foods high in fat, fiber, and protein right before exercise as they take longer to digest and may cause stomach upset.

Carbohydrates also play a crucial role in recovery. After a workout, muscle cells are most open to receiving carbohydrates and take up glucose like a sponge. Muscle cells are also more insulin sensitive after a workout, and insulin is key for glycogen synthesis. It is crucial for athletes to replenish muscle glycogen stores. It is like putting gas in your car: you never want to run on empty.

Athletes that have tough training sessions or competitions less than 8 hours apart should consume carbohydrates as soon as possible after exercise to maximize their recovery. It is recommended to consume 1 to 1.2 g of carbohydrate per kilogram per hour for the first 4 hours after exercise. For athletes that have longer recovery periods (24 hours or more), the timing and amount can be spread out more, as long as the athlete is meeting the carbohydrate and energy needs.

During sustained, high-intensity workouts lasting 30 to 75 minutes, consuming small amounts of carbohydrates can be helpful for enhancing performance. For endurance workouts lasting longer than an hour, it is wise to consume easily digestible carbohydrates during the workout. This can include drinks or snacks such as sports drinks, gels, gummies, and fruit. Popular, the many easily digestible intraworkout carbohydrate choices include sports drink, gels, gummies, and fruit.

The Role of Protein

Protein needs in athletes are greater than those of the average person, but intake need not be excessive. The major role of protein is to help repair, build, and strengthen muscles. Protein is also important for other things, such as keeping the immune system strong, growing nails and hair, and replacing red blood cells. Unlike carbohydrates, there is no storage form of protein. Any excess protein is converted and used for energy or stored as fat or glycogen as a last resort. Therefore, it is important that athletes consume protein daily, evenly distributed throughout the day.

In general, athletes require 1.2 to 2.0 g of protein per kilogram of body weight. It is best that protein is spread throughout the day. Most athletes should aim for a minimum of 20-25 g of protein at meals. This could easily be achieved by including eggs at breakfast, chicken at lunch, fish or lean red meat at dinner, and things such as yogurt, protein shakes, and chocolate milk as snacks. Vegan and vegetarian athletes need to carefully plan their meals to consume adequate protein. Plant-based protein is less bioavailable than animal-based protein, so protein needs in these athletes may be greater.

Plant-based diets are a hot topic in the general population and among athletes, although there is no real definition for plant based, which can be both confusing and misleading. Some people interpret it as a vegetarian or vegan diet, whereas others focus on adding more fruits and vegetables to their plates. Athletes deciding to go vegetarian or vegan must create a customized plan with their dietitians to make sure they are meeting their nutrition needs. These athletes are at greater risk of deficiency for the following nutrients:

- Protein
- Zinc
- Iron
- B_{12}
- Calcium

Major dietary changes (such as switching to a vegan/vegetarian diet) should only be made in the off-season so it does not negatively affect the athlete's energy, performance, and nutrition status during practice and competitions.

The Role of Fat

In sports, protein and carbohydrates get most of the attention. However, fat is a major source of fuel for athletes during light to moderate exercise intensities and long endurance exercise. Fat is also necessary for the absorption of fat-soluble vitamins A, D, E, and K. Athletes should not restrict their fat intakes because it can decrease diet quality and make it harder to reach their total energy needs, which can affect both performance and overall health. Fat restriction also limits essential fatty acids (especially the n-3 fatty acids) and fat-soluble phytonutrients.

In recent years, the ketogenic diet has been a topic of interest, especially in endurance sports. The ketogenic diet is a high-fat, very-low-carbohydrate diet that has the potential to induce ketosis. The first studies on the ketogenic diet came out in the

1930s for the treatment of epilepsy and were medically monitored. Over the last few years, it has regained popularity and is of particular interest to athletes as an ergogenic aid. In endurance sports, some studies suggest that following the ketogenic diet can help athletes prevent burnout when the body runs out of carbohydrates. By relying on fat for energy instead, it may help the athletes exercise longer. However, there is evidence that the lack of carbohydrates can decrease exercise intensity,[1] especially for athletes that perform at high intensity, or in sports that need access to quick energy, such as weight lifting or basketball. In elite race walkers, researchers found that, compared with diets with chronic or periodized high carbohydrate availability, the ketogenic diet impairs performance in part because of reduced exercise economy.[2]

Another consideration with the ketogenic diet is its effect on exercise recovery. A recent study of the effects of a non–energy-restricted ketogenic diet on muscle fatigue in young, healthy women found that the ketogenic diet had a negative effect on muscle fatigue both during daily activities and during exercise.[3]

Aside from any performance benefits, there is a real risk of nutrient and overall energy deficiencies in athletes following the ketogenic diet. It is extremely restrictive and difficult to sustain for a long period of time.

Energy Needs and Low Energy Availability

Adequate energy or calorie intake is essential for overall well-being and performance. When there are not enough calories being consumed to meet an athlete's needs, this is known as low energy availability (EA). This condition can lead to hormonal imbalances, depressed immunity status, bone disorders (such as low mineral density and stress fractures), gastrointestinal and cardiovascular dysfunction, and compromised psychological health.[4]

The prevalence of low EA in sports ranges from 22% to 58%, including both men and women.[5] For women, low energy intake, menstrual dysfunction, and low bone mineral density were widely recognized as the female athlete triad. However, in 2015 the International Olympic Committee introduced a revised term for this condition called relative energy deficiency in sport (RED-S). RED-S includes a larger scope of all related low-EA conditions and opens it up to both genders, not just women. Although less understood and studied in men, it is apparent that low EA exists, as shown by studies conducted in male cyclists[4] and endurance athletes.[6]

The origins of low EA are complex and must be addressed appropriately to avoid negative long-term health effects. Although some cases of low EA are a result of unintentional dietary intake, a more serious pattern of disordered eating or a clinical eating disorder may be the underlying cause.

The Low Energy Availability in Female Questionnaire (LEAF-Q) is a validated, 25-question screening tool that was developed to identify women at risk of low EA, abnormal reproductive function, and poor bone health. It is reported that a questionnaire for male athletes called the Low Energy Availability in Males Questionnaire is being developed.[7]

Disordered eating and eating disorders in athletes

Affecting about 9% of the population worldwide, eating disorders are serious and complex mental illnesses characterized by disturbances in eating and food-related behavior. They are among the deadliest mental illnesses, second only to opioid overdose.[8] Individuals with anorexia nervosa experience 6 times the mortality of their peers, whereas those with bulimia nervosa and atypical eating disorders have double the death rate of their nondisordered peers.[9]

Despite these statistics, many eating disorders unrecognized either because the individuals do not believe they are sick enough to warrant help, or because their behaviors are normalized and even praised in our diet-obsessed society. For athletes, they might not want to admit they have a problem for fear of being pulled out of their sports. Treatment of eating disorders ideally includes an experienced multidisciplinary team of medical, nutrition, and mental health professionals.

Feeding and Eating Disorders in the Diagnostic and Statistical Manual of Mental Disorders, Fifth Edition

Previously, eating disorders were divided into 3 major subgroups: anorexia nervosa, bulimia nervosa, and eating disorder not otherwise specified (EDNOS). More recently, the Diagnostic and Statistical Manual of Mental Disorders, Fifth Edition (DSM-5) eliminated EDNOS and expanded to include pica, rumination disorder, avoidant/restrictive food intake disorder (ARFID), binge-eating disorder, other specified feeding or eating disorder (OSFED), and unspecified feeding or eating disorder . These changes have significantly changed clinicians' ability to officially diagnose and provide earlier and more specific clinical interventions. Less commonly known feeding and eating disorders in the DSM-5 include:

ARFID: problem with eating unrelated to weight or shape concerns, leading to the inability to meet nutrition needs
Pica: recurrent consumption of nonnutritive, nonfood items such as clay, paint, paper
Rumination disorder: recurrent, effortless regurgitation of food that may be re-chewed, reswallowed, or spat out

In addition to the expanded list of feeding and eating disorders, the DSM-5 includes a Comorbidity section. Although not extensive, it addresses many of the other common psychiatric diagnoses associated with the particular eating and feeding disorders. For example, anxiety disorders, higher-than-expected rates of substance abuse, and major depressive disorder are commonly seen in anorexia nervosa. Note that mood changes that have physiologic and psychological causes are highly affected by calorie restriction and weights below threshold. Weight restoration and nutritional rehabilitation are of paramount importance in these cases, and only once the persons are no longer in a starved state are they able to fully benefit from therapy (medicinal and otherwise).

Similarly, patients with binge-eating disorder and bulimia nervosa have a high rate of major depression and substance use disorder. Patients with bulimia nervosa have high rates of suicidality and posttraumatic stress disorder (37%). Depression is the most common comorbid psychiatric disorder for individuals with binge-eating disorder along with high rates of anxiety disorders, specifically panic disorder and simple phobia.[10]

Although the criteria for the various feeding and eating disorders are outlined in the DSM-5, some presentations of eating disorders are less obvious. Any patient with restrictive thoughts about weight or shape or abnormal behaviors around food warrants the consideration for an eating disorder diagnosis. For example, a study of more than 4000 women aged 25 to 45 years found that approximately 70% of the women engaged in disordered eating behaviors without a history of an eating disorder. An alarming 75% of women reported that their concerns about shape and weight interfered with their happiness. Disordered eating is widely prevalent and can have serious mental and physical consequences. It is important to take these signs seriously.

However, behaviors that accompany disordered eating are so common that they are often normalized and accepted by peers, parents, medical professionals, and coaches. Most people would not think twice about a friend following a Paleo diet or intermittent fasting. In fact, they are often praised for their will power and dedication. It is common to hear people talk about a cupcake being bad or a salad being good, or how they are going to "run off" that pizza they just ate tomorrow.

One of the most obvious signs of disordered eating is dieting, but it also includes behaviors that reflect eating disorders such as anorexia nervosa, bulimia nervosa, binge-eating disorder, or OSFED. **Box 1** lists some signs of disordered eating.

Who Is at Risk?

Historically, eating disorders were associated with young, heterosexual, white women. However, eating disorders can affect anyone, regardless of age, gender identity, race, socioeconomic status, or body weight or size. Despite similar rates of eating disorder symptoms across ethnic groups, people of color who acknowledged their struggles with food and weight were less likely to be asked about eating disorder symptoms by their doctors.[11] Food insecurity is a big risk factor for the development of an eating disorder: about 17% of people using American food banks have clinically significant eating disorder symptoms.[12] Experiencing food scarcity or not having access to enough food can have a negative impact on people's mental health and their relationships with food.

Eating disorders and body image issues exist across all gender identities. Disordered eating behaviors among men are nearly just as common as they are among women. About 1 in 3 people with an eating disorder is male. Research suggests that transgender people are more likely than cisgender people to have been diagnosed with an eating disorder or to engage in disordered eating.[13] More studies

---

Box 1
Signs of disordered eating

1. Food is considered to be good" or bad
   For example: "These cookies are so bad; I shouldn't be eating them!" Or, "I'll be good today and have a salad." Athletes may even hear this from parents, peers, or coaches. They may think they are judged or not committed enough for eating certain foods. Food shaming is all too common in society and can often lead to restriction, sneak eating, or other disordered behaviors.

2. Not trusting oneself around certain foods
   For example: "I don't keep cereal in the house; I'll definitely overdo it."

3. Thinking about food all of the time
   For example: while eating breakfast, to already be thinking about what to eat for lunch. Or, during a breakfast meeting, thinking only about the bagels on the table. Planning and thinking about food takes up a lot of time, often making the person anxious.

4. Choosing lots of sugar-free or diet versions of food to save calories
   For example: filling cabinets with sugar-free pudding, low-carbohydrate tortillas, or GG crackers.

5. Unrealistic body expectations
   For example: people thinking that their thighs are never thin enough or stomach is never flat enough. Or maybe their muscles are not big enough or "ripped" enough. Various forms of body checking, including zeroing in on certain body parts, weighing themselves frequently, comparing their bodies with others, and skin pinching, occur often in people with disordered eating and eating disorders.

need to be done to determine the prevalence of eating disorders or disordered eating across the gender identity spectrum.

One of the biggest misconceptions about eating disorders is that there is a particular "look" or that everyone that struggles with an eating disorder is underweight. It is important to understand that eating disorders can happen at *any* weight and any body size. Less than 6% of people with eating disorders are medically diagnosed as underweight.[14]

Athletes are no less vulnerable to eating disorders. A large study found that clinical or subclinical eating disorders were more prevalent in athletes than in the general population.[15] Eating disorders are most prominent in sports that focus on leanness and weight. About 40% to 42% of women in aesthetic sports and 30% to 35% of women in weight class sports have eating disorders. For male athletes, about 17% to 18% in weight class and 22% to 42% in gravitational sports have eating disorders.[16]

In addition to sociocultural pressures to achieve and maintain the ideal body type, athletes are also under pressure to improve performance and conform to the requirements of their sports. Athletes are constantly subjected to comments and thoughts about their body compositions and shapes, especially in sports such as dance or figure skating. They tend to trust in their coaches and trainers, who offer nutrition advice despite a lack of formal training in this area. Their drive to please and excel may lead to use of extreme weight-control methods and eating behaviors. **Box 2** presents risk factors for an eating disorder in athletes.

Medical and Psychological Considerations

Although athletes are at risk for all the same medical complications that result from an eating disorder, they are at a higher risk for things such as stress fractures and electrolyte disturbances, depending on the sport. **Box 3** presents common medical complications related to eating disorders.

There are several personality traits and vulnerabilities that have been identified that put athletes at increased risk of developing an eating disorder. Perfectionism was found to be a significant predictor of disordered eating risk in male and female elite soccer players.[17] In female athletes specifically, disordered eating seems to be influenced by perfectionism, competitiveness, pain tolerance, and the perceived performance advantage of weight loss.[18] Other psychological risk factors include

---

Box 2
Risk factors for an eating disorder in athletes

- Sports that emphasize appearance or require competitors to make weight. For example, gymnastics, diving, wrestling, body building

- Sports that focus on individuals rather than an entire team; for example, figure skating, dance, and diving

- Antigravity sports; for example, ski-jumping or other jumping events

- Endurance sports, such as swimming or track and field

- Inaccurate belief that a lower weight will improve performance

- Low self-esteem; family dysfunction; families with eating disorders; chronic dieting; history of physical or sexual abuse; peer, family, and cultural pressures to be thin; and other traumatic life experiences

- Athletes who become injured and think they need to cut back on their food intake despite increased nutritional needs for healing

obsessionality, social anxiety, shyness, excessive compliance, and low self-esteem.[19] The two most prevalent personality disorders among individuals with eating disorders seem to be obsessive-compulsive disorder (anorexia nervosa, restricting type) and borderline personality disorder (anorexia nervosa, binge-eating purging type; bulimia nervosa).[20]

Having a high athletic identity is thought to increase vulnerability for compulsive exercise and eating disorder behavior. Brewer and colleagues[21] describe athletic identity as the degree to which an individual identifies with the athlete role and looks to others for acknowledgment of that role. Although there are some benefits to having a strong athletic identity (strong sense of self, self-confidence, possibly enhanced performance), there may be some negative psychological consequences (emotional difficulties during injury, difficulty adjusting to life after the end of the athletic career). When an athlete's self-worth and identity are tightly tied into the role as an athlete, anything that challenges that can increase the athlete's vulnerability to eating disorder triggers (eg, low self-esteem, weight/shape concerns, critical comments).[22]

Early detection and treatment of eating disorders

Eating disorders have harmful effects on the health and performance of athletes. Athletes, parents, coaches, athletic administrators, sports psychologists, and team doctors are all important players in eating disorder prevention. If an athlete is showing any warning signs of an eating disorder, this should be taken seriously. Early detection increases the likelihood of successful treatment. **Box 4** presents the warning signs of an eating disorder.

In assessing a patient with a suspected eating disorder, a comprehensive history and physical examination should be completed. There are several eating disorder screening tools that may be useful, including The SCOFF (Sick, Control, One, Fat, Food) questionnaire, The Brief Eating Disorders in Athletes Questionnaire, The Athletic Milieu Direct Questionnaire, and The Female Athlete Screening Tool.[23]

In addition to common history questions, athletes should be asked about their current eating patterns, body image, weight-control measures, and how often they exercise, and psychiatric conditions should be assessed. If the primary care provider is the

---

Box 3
Common medical complications related to eating disorders

- Electrolyte and fluid disturbances
- Lanugo
- Gastroparesis
- Constipation
- Hormonal disturbances
- Bone density loss
- Decreased white blood cell count
- Cardiac abnormalities
- Hair changes/loss
- Acrocyanosis
- Low blood pressure
- Dehydration

Box 4
Warning signs of an eating disorder

- Intense fear of gaining weight
- Refusal to eat or highly restrictive eating
- Frequent dieting
- Compulsive exercise or rigid exercise routines
- Sensitivity to cold
- Absent or irregular menstrual periods in women
- Hair loss
- Body dysmorphia
- Excessive facial or body hair
- Withdrawal from friends and family
- Evidence of binge eating
- Frequent trips to the bathroom after eating
- Feeling guilt or shame after eating

---

first to suspect or diagnose an eating disorder, the provider can then help the athlete formulate a treatment team. An eating disorder dietitian and psychologist are crucial members of this team.

In some cases, athletes may be pulled out of their sports because it is not medically safe to exercise. That decision is at the discretion of the treatment team and is managed on a case-by-case basis. For children and adolescents, caregivers should also be interviewed and included in the treatment plan. When feasible, treatment protocols have shifted away from individualized therapy for most adolescents and young adults, to family-based therapy. Family-based therapy is now seen as the gold standard and most effective for the treatment of anorexia nervosa and bulimia nervosa.[24] This therapeutic approach places parental (or guardian) involvement at the center of care. Full recovery is difficult without a strong support system. If the athlete is medically unstable or psychiatrically unstable, a comprehensive multidisciplinary treatment

---

Box 5
Useful tips in managing athletes with eating disorders

- Instill hope. This time is stressful and scary for the athletes and for their family members or caregivers. Full recovery is possible.
- Eating disorders are mental illnesses that best respond to weight restoration and normalization of eating behaviors.
- Target behaviors. In some cases, weight restoration is the most important thing to focus on. For others, it may be other behaviors, such as purging.
- Treatment should not be delayed. Eating disorders can become chronic, so getting a qualified treatment team in place is of utmost importance.
- Consult with trained specialists with experience caring for athletes with eating disorders. Referring to someone who does not have the qualifications to treat eating disorders can delay recovery. This point is more important than who is most convenient to see.

---

plan is indicated; **Box 5** presents useful tips in managing athletes with eating disorders.

SUMMARY

Sports nutrition has grown over recent years. Athletes are actively seeking out fueling tactics and nutrition recommendations to give them a competitive advantage; they are often driven by influence from coaches, teammates, athletic trainers, and even social media. There is also the influence of the multibillion-dollar diet industry selling supplements, diet plans, energy drinks, proteins bars, and other aids. Food fads, such as gluten free and keto, and catchy phrases such as clean eating and plant based can lead to confusion about what healthy eating is for athletes. This confusion can lead to overly restrictive eating, chronic underfueling, disordered eating behaviors, or full-blown eating disorders. It is important to recognize the signs of disordered eating in athletes and understand that an eating disorder can occur across all genders, all sports, and at any weight or body size. Sports nutritionists play an important role in recognizing issues related to nutrition and helping to develop strategies that maximize performance.

REFERENCES

1. Zajac A, Poprzecki S, Maszczyk A, et al. The effects of a ketogenic diet on exercise metabolism and physical performance in off-road cyclists. Nutrients 2014;6: 2493–508.
2. Burke LM, Ross ML, Garvican-Lewis LA, et al. Low carbohydrate, high fat diet impairs exercise economy and negates the performance benefit from intensified training in elite race walkers. J Physiol 2017;595:2785–807.
3. Sjödin A, Hellström F, Sehlstedt E, et al. Effects of a ketogenic diet on muscle fatigue in healthy, young, normal-weight women: a randomized controlled feeding trial. Nutrients 2020;12:955.
4. Logue DM, Madigan SM, Melin A, et al. Low energy availability in athletes 2020: an updated narrative review of prevalence, risk, within-day energy balance, knowledge, and impact on sports performance. Nutrients 2020;12:835.
5. Burke LM, Close GL, Lundy B, et al. Relative energy deficiency in sport in male athletes: a commentary on its presentation among selected groups of male athletes. Int J Sport Nutr Exerc Metab 2018;28:364–74.
6. Torstveit MK, Fahrenholtz IL, Lichtenstein MB, et al. Exercise dependence, eating disorder symptoms and biomarkers of relative energy deficiency in sports (RED-S) among male endurance athletes. BMJ Open Sport Exerc Med 2019;5: e000439.
7. Mountjoy M, Sundgot-Borgen JK, Burke LM, et al. IOC consensus statement on relative energy deficiency in sport (RED-S): 2018 update. Br J Sports Med 2018;52:687–97.
8. Chesney E, Goodwin GM, Fazel S. Risks of all-cause and suicide mortality in mental disorders: a meta-review. World Psych 2014;13:153–60.
9. Arcelus J, Mitchell AJ, Wales J, et al. Mortality rates in patients with anorexia nervosa and other eating disorders. A meta-analysis of 36 studies. Arch Gen Psychiatry 2011;68:724–31.
10. Mitchell JE, Wonderlich SA. Feeding and eating disorders. In: Hales RE, Yudofsky SC, Roberts LW, editors. The American Psychiatric Publishing textbook of psychiatry. American Psychiatric Publishing, Inc; 2014. p. 557–86.

11. Becker AE, Franko DL, Speck A, et al. Ethnicity and differential access to care for eating disorder symptoms. Int J Eat Disord 2003;33:205–12.
12. Becker CB, Middlemass KM, Gomez F, et al. Eating disorder pathology among individuals living with food insecurity: a replication study. Clin Psychol Sci 2019;7:1144–58.
13. Diemer EW, Grant JD, Munn-Chernoff MA, et al. Gender identity, sexual orientation, and eating-related pathology in a national sample of college students. J Adolesc Health 2015;57:144–9.
14. Flament MF, Henderson K, Buchholz A, et al. Weight status and DSM-5 diagnoses of eating disorders in adolescents from the community. J Am Acad Child Adolesc Psychiatry 2015;54:403–11.e2.
15. Sundgot-Borgen J, Torstveit MK. Prevalence of eating disorders in elite athletes is higher than in the general population. Clin J Sport Med 2004;14:25–32.
16. Sundgot-Borgen J, Torstveit MK. Aspects of disordered eating continuum in elite high-intensity sports. Scand J Med Sci Sports 2010;20:112–21.
17. Abbott W, Brett A, Brownlee TE, et al. The prevalence of disordered eating in elite male and female soccer players. Eat Weight Disord 2021;26(2):491–8.
18. Stirling A, Kerr G. Perceived vulnerabilities of female athletes to the development of disordered eating behaviours. Eur J Sport Sci 2012;12:262–73.
19. Fairburn CG, Cooper Z, Doll HA, et al. Risk factors for anorexia nervosa: three integrated case-control comparisons. Arch Gen Psychiatry 1999;56:468–76.
20. Sansone RA, Sansone LA. Personality pathology and its influence on eating disorders. Innov Clin Neurosci 2011;8:14–8.
21. Brewer BW, Van Raalte JL, Linder DE. Athletic identity: Hercules' muscles or Achilles heel? Internat J Sport Psychol 1993;24:237–54.
22. Turton R, Goodwin H, Meyer C. Athletic identity, compulsive exercise and eating psychopathology in long-distance runners. Eat Behav 2017;26:129–32.
23. Morgan JF, Reid F, Lacey JH. The SCOFF questionnaire: assessment of a new screening tool for eating disorders. BMJ 1999;319:1467–8.
24. Lock J, Le Grange D, Agras WS, et al. Randomized clinical trial comparing family-based treatment with adolescent-focused individual therapy for adolescents with anorexia nervosa. Arch Gen Psychiatry 2010;67:1025–32.

Pathophysiology of Traumatic Brain Injury, Chronic Traumatic Encephalopathy, and Neuropsychiatric Clinical Expression

Sharon Baughman Shively, MD, PhD[a], David S. Priemer, MD[b,c], Murray B. Stein, MD, MPH[d,e], Daniel P. Perl, MD[f,*]

KEYWORDS

- Traumatic brain injury (TBI) • Chronic traumatic encephalopathy (CTE)
- Posttraumatic stress disorder (PTSD) • Dementia • Tauopathy

KEY POINTS

- Chronic traumatic encephalopathy (CTE) is presently considered to be a tauopathy, associated with multiple mild impact traumatic brain injuries (TBIs) from events such as contact sports, domestic violence and head banging, or possibly with single moderate or severe TBI from an event such as a motor vehicle accident.
- CTE diagnosis currently can only be rendered with neuropathological examination of the brain at autopsy, with no definitive antemortem signs/symptoms or established in vivo biomarkers for validated diagnostics or effective therapy.
- Nonspecific behavioral, mood, cognitive and motor changes, which vary among individuals, may be associated with CTE.
- CTE may share clinical features with and neuroanatomic sites implicated in posttraumatic stress disorder.
- Current data point to the glymphatic pathway for homeostatic clearance of fluids and proteins, possibly including the deleterious protein p-tau. The glymphatic clearance of p-tau in the extracellular space from damaged axons due to TBI, as well as local neuron and astrocyte uptake, may explain the signature p-tau pattern of CTE in the human neocortex.

---

[a] Independent Researcher, Potomac, MD, USA; [b] F. Edward Hébert School of Medicine, Uniformed Services University of the Health Sciences, Bethesda, MD, USA; [c] Henry M. Jackson Foundation for the Advancement of Military Medicine, Bethesda, MD, USA; [d] University of California San Diego, La Jolla, CA, USA; [e] Veterans Affairs San Diego Healthcare System, La Jolla, CA, USA; [f] Department of Pathology, F. Edward Hébert School of Medicine, Uniformed Services University of the Health Sciences, 4301 Jones Bridge Road, Room B-3138, Bethesda, MD 20814, USA
* Corresponding author.
E-mail address: daniel.perl@usuhs.edu

Psychiatr Clin N Am 44 (2021) 443–458
https://doi.org/10.1016/j.psc.2021.04.003
0193-953X/21/© 2021 Elsevier Inc. All rights reserved.

INTRODUCTION

Chronic traumatic encephalopathy (CTE) evolved from observations of clinical and neuropathological sequelae after repeated mild impact traumatic brain injuries (TBIs) in boxers. In 1928, American pathologist Harrison Martland[1] originally put forth the concept that boxers with repeated head injury could suffer from a debilitating medical condition, initially called "punch drunk." He described boxers as often showing symptoms of staggering, disequilibrium, mental confusion, slowed muscular movement or appearing intoxicated. Years after retirement, some boxers displayed signs of parkinsonism and/or cognitive dysfunction. Martland[1] urged the medical community to establish or refute the existence of punch drunk as a clinical entity by comparing antemortem neurologic examinations with postmortem neuropathological studies. Approximately 3 decades later, Macdonald Critchley[2,3] further studied and comprehensively illustrated numerous clinical phenotypes associated with the punch drunk state and first used the term CTE with specific reference to boxers who had developed neurologic signs/symptoms after a prolonged period of latency. At the time of Critchley's[2,3] reporting, only 1 autopsy study of a former boxer's brain had been reported.[4] In the 1960s, from the study of 224 retired British boxers while focusing on motor abnormalities, Anthony Roberts[5] acknowledged the wide spectrum of clinical presentations among individuals, ranging from mild forms with dysarthria, asymmetric pyramidal lesions, and disequilibrium, to severe disability with ataxias, rigidity, tremor, and dementia. Eventually, the term CTE extended to athletes in contact sports with inherent risk of mild TBIs (concussions) or subconcussive injuries, and additionally to other situations with potential repetitive head injuries such as domestic violence, head banging or poorly controlled epilepsy.[6]

Within the past 2 decades, a surge of interest in CTE has led to advancement in our understanding of the disease, with particular respect to neuropathologic observations and classification, but also in characterizing symptomology and theorizing pathophysiology. However, the reported signs and symptoms of CTE are nonspecific, and the described neuropathologic features of CTE have yet to be sufficiently correlated with the broad spectrum and varied severity of those clinical features. The specificity of the recently designated neuropathologic features of CTE is also a subject of recent controversy. In addition, the general population is not adequately represented in CTE research, as the large majority focused on individuals in contact sports, especially on the professional level. Ultimately, although CTE has received much recent media attention, which would otherwise suggest that the medical community has fully characterized the illness, there are currently many substantial gaps in our knowledge of the condition.

CHRONIC TRAUMATIC ENCEPHALOPATHY CLINICAL FEATURES

CTE is currently designated a tauopathy, distinct from neurodegenerative diseases involving the abnormal hyperphosphorylation of the endogenous protein tau (p-tau) such as Alzheimer disease and some forms of frontotemporal dementia (eg, Pick disease). As aforementioned, CTE pathology is classically described in association with history of repeated mild TBIs from contact sports, but also in association with other circumstances of repetitive impact head injury, such as domestic violence, head banging, or poorly controlled epilepsy. CTE is also classically characterized by a period of latency between initial injuries and symptom presentation, which is often many years in duration, with a clinical onset typically ranging from the second to seventh decades of life.[7] However, the reported symptoms of CTE are nonspecific and as of today antemortem methods of CTE diagnosis have yet to be developed that carefully and reliably delineate CTE from the clinical presentations of other disorders (eg, other dementing illnesses, primary psychiatric disease, substance abuse). Although this difficulty largely exists for most proteinopathies that, to this date, require postmortem examination for definitive diagnosis, CTE is relatively unique among the neurodegenerative proteinopathies, in that it may not inherently be a clinically progressive disorder. CTE neuropsychiatric abnormalities can exacerbate and expand with time in some patients,[8] which has been associated with extensive accumulation of p-tau in the human brain at autopsy; however, clinical progression with burgeoning p-tau deposition leading to advanced CTE stages may not occur in all cases.[9,10] Examples of prominent behavioral and mood features, often formerly uncharacteristic to the person, include explosive rage, depression, anxiety, irritability, impulsivity, apathy, and paranoia.[9,10] Other common complaints include headache, difficulty sleeping, memory impairment, poor concentration, reduced capacity to make decisions, visuospatial problems and language difficulties. Dementia and parkinsonism may also develop. Possibly in congruence with cognitive and mood/behavioral dysfunctions, in anecdotal instances patients who have been found to have CTE pathology were noted to have suffered deterioration in interpersonal relationships (eg, spousal abuse, divorce), indulged in criminal and violent behavior, displayed dismal money management leading to bankruptcy, experienced diminished social status, and developed substance abuse. Not infrequently, patients also have committed suicide or died as a consequence of engaging in poorly conceived, high-risk behaviors commonly deemed as accidents (including drug overdoses).

As mentioned, the clinical features ascribed to CTE are often nonspecific; well-designed, controlled studies that clinically delineate CTE from other conditions have not been performed. And so, although the medical literature outlines signs and symptoms associated with neuropathological features for CTE, evidence-based diagnostic criteria based on correlation to pathologic findings and understanding of underlying pathophysiology, do not currently exist. Although research efforts including those to ascertain neuroimaging modalities and other biomarkers for the living are ongoing, a diagnosis of CTE can presently only be rendered with postmortem examination of the brain. As such, clinicians currently must rely on patient history of TBI in conjunction with presentation of neuropsychiatric symptoms, which may indicate underlying CTE neuropathology.

CLINICAL OVERLAP OF POSTTRAUMATIC STRESS DISORDER AND CHRONIC TRAUMATIC ENCEPHALOPATHY

The pathophysiology after TBI and biological underpinnings of CTE potentially affect psychiatric symptom expression within specific diagnoses established in the *Diagnostic and Statistical Manual of Mental Disorders, 5th Edition: DSM-5*. One complex example is PTSD, for which *DSM* authors have continuously recommended consideration of TBI in the clinical evaluation ever since the introduction of PTSD as a clinical entity with the *DSM-III* publication in 1980. For a diagnosis of PTSD according to *DSM-5*, a patient presents with clinical features satisfying 8 categories of symptomatology (Criteria A–H).[11] Symptoms associated with CTE can overlap with, and thus partially fulfill the diagnostic requirements for PTSD (**Table 1**). In addition, in some cases of PTSD, patients live for years before development of symptoms sufficient for diagnosis, known as delayed expression, which complements concepts in CTE such as latency (time between TBI and symptom onset) and potential expansion and exacerbation of symptoms over time. Nonetheless, CTE symptomatology does not fulfill Criterion B of the PTSD diagnostic criteria, which requires the presence of one intrusion symptom,

Table 1
Patients with CTE can express clinical features that partially satisfy criteria for PTSD diagnosis according to *DSM-5*

PTSD Criteria (*DSM-5*, See Original Text for Full Detail)	Overlap Between CTE and PTSD
Criterion A: exposure to actual or threatened death, serious injury or sexual violence in at least 1 of 4 ways (A1-A4)	*Criterion A1*: directly experiencing the traumatic event(s) (History of TBI, dependent on circumstance)
Criterion B: at least 1 of 5 intrusion symptoms associated with the traumatic event(s) (B1-B5)	None
Criterion C: at least 1 of 2 symptoms indicating persistent avoidance of stimuli associated with the traumatic event(s) (C1-C2)	None
Criterion D: at least 2 of 7 symptoms indicating negative alterations in cognitions and mood associated with the traumatic events(s), beginning or worsening after the traumatic event(s) (D1-D7)	*Criterion D1:* inability to remember an important aspect of the traumatic event(s), typically due to dissociative amnesia and not to other factors such as head injury, alcohol, or drugs (with absent TBI history, patient could fulfill criterion due to altered consciousness or posttraumatic amnesia) *Criterion D5:* Markedly diminished interest or participation in significant activities
Criterion E: at least 2 of 6 symptoms indicating marked alterations in arousal and reactivity associated with the traumatic event(s), beginning or worsening after the traumatic event(s) (E1-E6)	*Criterion E1*: Irritable behavior and angry outbursts (with little or no provocation) typically expressed as verbal or physical aggression toward people or objects *Criterion E2*: Reckless or self-destructive behavior *Criterion E5*: Problems with concentration *Criterion E6*: Sleep disturbance
Criterion F: duration of disturbance (Criteria B, C, D, E) more than 1 mo	Long-term persistence of symptomology, with progressive exacerbation and expansion of clinical symptoms in some cases
Criterion G: disturbance causes clinically significant distress or impairment in social, occupational or other important areas of functioning	Headache, motor abnormalities, poor social and family relationships, diminished socioeconomic status
Criterion H: disturbance not attributable to physiologic effects of a substance or another medical condition	CTE not clinically defined well enough to qualify as definitive alternative medical condition; however, some patients currently diagnosed with TBI and PTSD

Abbreviations: CTE, chronic traumatic encephalopathy; PTSD, posttraumatic stress disorder; TBI, traumatic brain injury.
Data from McKee AC, Stein TD, Nowinski CJ, et al. The spectrum of disease in chronic traumatic encephalopathy. Brain 2013;136(Pt 1):43-64.

or Criterion C, which requires 1 symptom indicating persistent avoidance of stimuli associated with the traumatic event(s).

The literature addressing CTE clinical expression mostly incorporates athletes from contact sports, and largely does not control for additional history of psychotraumatic event(s) either before, during or after the TBI incident(s), which may ultimately influence symptomatology. Therefore, the superimposition of TBI history and psychotraumatic experiences may complicate the diagnosis of PTSD and/or the clinical consideration of CTE. It may also be possible that the structural or functional alterations from CTE (or TBI in general) may compromise neurocircuits necessary to cope with the psychotraumatic experience, thereby promoting the possibility of PTSD development, although this is a matter of ongoing controversy. Pointedly, CTE cases with antemortem PTSD clinical history have been reported, particularly in the military[9] but the degree to which CTE may have contributed to the PTSD symptomatology clinically remains uncertain. Also of interest, recent literature suggests that individuals diagnosed with PTSD have higher risk for manifesting clinical dementia, in both military and general populations.[12,13] Although study patient cohorts tend to be heterogeneous (and do not necessarily address TBI history), these papers further hint at an association among TBI, PTSD, and dementia (possibly including CTE cases). For example, one salient study with prospective and retrospective analytical components showed frontotemporal dementia as the most common clinical phenotype among the patients with dementia of the PTSD clinical cohorts, which were derived from the general population.[14] Frontotemporal dementia symptoms can clinically resemble those of CTE, and similarly this disease necessitates autopsy for definitive diagnosis. This particular study did not provide TBI history or confirmation of clinical phenotype with autopsy findings, resultantly not excluding the possibility of CTE as an underlying form of dementia in these cases. In summary, there is some clinical overlap between symptoms of CTE/TBI and PTSD, and this may complicate their diagnoses. In superimposed circumstances, the degree to which they each may influence similar symptomatology is also uncertain.

CHRONIC TRAUMATIC ENCEPHALOPATHY NEUROPATHOLOGY

Akin to other tauopathies, CTE entails abnormal p-*tau* accumulation within neurons (known as neurofibrillary tangles or NFTs, **Fig. 1**D) and astrocytes.[9] Endogenous *tau* protein normally resides within axons, stabilizing neuronal microtubules to aid with transport of essential components necessary for cell survival and function (**Fig. 1**A). In neurodegenerative disease, *tau* protein gains phosphate groups, disassociates from microtubules, undergoes conformational change and aggregates in insoluble form (**Fig. 1**B,C). With normal aging, minimal p-*tau* aggregates can be identified in the medial temporal lobe, as early as 14 years of age.[15–17] Neurofibrillary changes beyond the medial temporal lobe, or otherwise widespread, indicate tauopathy other than aging, especially in young persons.[17,18]

More than 4 decades after Martland's[1] call for clinicopathological studies, Corsellis and colleagues[19] reported results of postmortem brain examinations from 15 retired boxers, with corresponding patient clinical histories. The study revealed patterns of mild cerebral atrophy, enlarged lateral ventricles with fenestrated cavum septum pellucidum, atrophied fornices detaching from a thinned corpus callosum, and cerebellar scarring. The investigators noted neuronal loss and NFTs spread diffusely in the cortices, hippocampus, and substantia nigra. They also correlated a subset of clinical symptoms with neuropathological findings, such as memory loss with hippocampus/ temporal lobe abnormalities and parkinsonism with NFTs in the substantia nigra. They

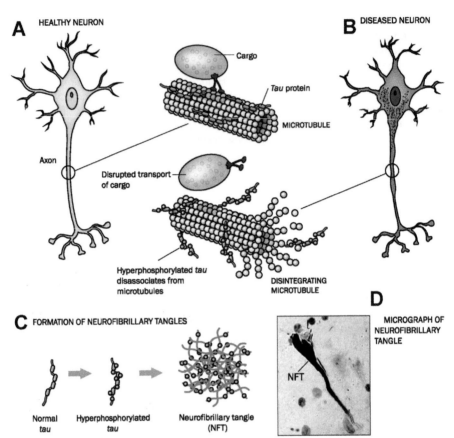

Fig. 1. (*A*) The endogenous brain protein *tau* normally binds microtubules within neuronal axons for stable transport of cargo with molecules necessary for cell viability and function. (*B*) In tauopathic disease (and axonal injury), *tau* gains phosphate groups and dissociates from microtubules, disrupting cargo transport and compromising cell function/viability. (*C*) Hyperphosphorylated *tau* (p-*tau*) forms insoluble aggregates within brain cells, including neurons (neurofibrillary tangles, NFTs). (*D*) Micrograph of p-*tau* immunoreactivity in a neuron (NFT).

admitted difficulty, however, in specifying anatomic sites accounting for symptoms such as outbursts of rage or aggression.

With the primary goal of differentiating CTE from other tauopathies, a consensus panel of neuropathology experts recently agreed on a pathognomonic lesion for CTE: accumulations of p-*tau* in neurons (NFTs), astrocytes (astrocytic tangles) and cell processes (p-*tau* immunoreactive neurites) distributed around small blood vessels at sulcal depths in irregular cortical spatial patterns.[6] This pathognomonic lesion is required for CTE diagnosis (**Fig. 2**B,D). Supportive diagnostic features were also described (**Table 2**) and largely included other p-*tau*-related findings that contrast with patterns of p-*tau* deposition in other tauopathies. For example, pretangles, NFTs, and/or extracellular tangles preferentially affecting superficial cortical layers II-III (as opposed to deeper layers)[20] and preferential involvement of p-*tau* in the CA2 and CA4 segments of the hippocampus and particular subcortical structures

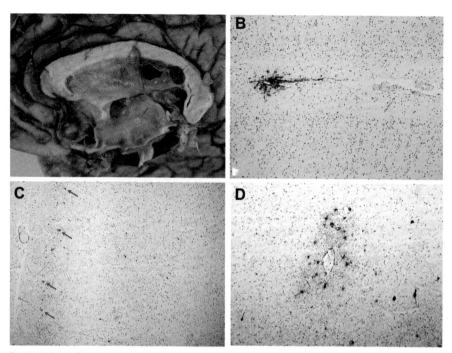

Fig. 2. Selected neuropathological features of CTE. (*A*) Mid-sagittal section of gross brain showing fenestrations in septum pellucidum. (*B*) P-*tau* immunoreactivity in neocortical brain tissue sample showing CTE pathognomonic lesion, defined as p-*tau* accumulations in neurons, astrocytes and cell processes distributed around small blood vessels at sulcal depths. (*C*) P-*tau* immunoreactivity in neocortical brain tissue sample showing NFTs (*arrows*) preferentially accumulating in superficial layers II-III. (*D*) Neocortical brain tissue sample showing perivascular p-*tau* immunoreactive neurons, astrocytes and cell processes.

(eg, mammillary bodies), support a diagnosis of CTE and are distinct from patterns of Alzheimer disease (**Fig. 2**C). The investigators additionally characterized common macroscopic findings as supportive diagnostic features, such as disproportionate dilatation of the third ventricle and septum pellucidum abnormalities (**Fig. 2**A).

McKee and colleagues[9] have extensively studied CTE postmortem brains, predominantly from former college and professional American football players, with associated clinical histories. By examining primarily hemispheric, 50-μm-thick, frozen coronal tissue sections, the clinical researchers proposed a neuropathological staging system for CTE, from stage I (mild) to stage IV (severe) based on density and regional deposition of p-*tau*.[9] In a second paper, the investigators further refined the staging system and provided data supporting positive associations among p-*tau* extent, advanced age, dementia and years of American football play.[21] The 4 stages are based on the extent and distribution of p-*tau* deposition and are as follows:

- Stage I. One or 2 foci of pathognomonic lesions, most commonly in frontal cortex; sparse NFTs in locus coeruleus.
- Stage II. Three or more foci of pathognomonic lesions in cortices of multiple lobes; NFTs in superficial neocortical layers (II-III), locus coeruleus, nucleus basalis of Meynert.

Table 2
CTE supportive neuropathological features according to the NINDS/NIBIB consensus meeting[4]

1. Pathognomonic neuropathological feature of CTE: p-*tau* accumulations in neurons, astrocytes, and cell processes distributed around small blood vessels at sulcal depths

2. Supportive neuropathological features of CTE:

p-*tau*-related pathology	non-p-*tau*-related pathology
i. Pretangles and NFTs in superficial cortical layers (II-III)	i. TDP-43 immunoreactive neuronal cytoplasmic inclusions and dot-like structures: hippocampus, anteromedial temporal cortex, amygdala
ii. Pretangles, NFTs or extracellular tangles preferentially involving CA2 of the hippocampus, and pretangles and prominent proximal dendritic swellings in CA4	ii. Macroscopic features:
iii. P-*tau* accumulation in neurons and astrocytes within subcortical nuclei (including mammillary bodies, hypothalamus, amygdala, nucleus accumbens, thalamus, midbrain tegmentum) and isodendritic core (including nucleus basalis of Meynert, raphe nuclei, substantia nigra, locus coeruleus)	• Disproportionate dilatation of the third ventricles relative to the lateral ventricles • Septal abnormalities (eg, cavum septum pellucidum, fenestrations/perforations) • Atrophy of the mammillary bodies • Signs of previous traumatic injury (eg, contusions)
iv. Thorny astrocytes at the glial limitans (most commonly in the subpial and periventricular regions) with p-*tau* immunoreactivity	
v. Large, grainlike and dot-like structures, in addition to thread-like neurites, with p-*tau* immunoreactivity	

Abbreviations: CA, Cornu ammonis; CTE, chronic traumatic encephalopathy; NFT, neurofibrillary tangles; NIBIB, National Institute of Biomedical Imaging and Bioengineering; NINDS, National Institute of Neurological Disorders and Stroke; PTSD, posttraumatic stress disorder; TDP-43, transactive response DNA binding protein 43 kDa.

- Stage III. Pathognomonic lesions in cortices of multiple lobes, often with larger clusters of p-*tau* at sulcal depths; NFTs in superficial neocortical layers (II-III), limbic system (hippocampus, entorhinal and perirhinal cortices, amygdala, thalamus, hypothalamus), substantia nigra, locus coeruleus, nucleus basalis of Meynert.
- Stage IV. Pathognomonic lesions in cortices of multiple lobes; NFTs throughout neocortex; severe neurofibrillary degeneration and associated neuron loss and gliosis in frontal and temporal cortices (particularly medial temporal lobe), diencephalon (including mammillary bodies), brainstem; NFTs in cerebellar dentate, basis pontis, spinal cord; macroscopic changes including generalized cerebral atrophy (most pronounced in frontal and temporal lobes especially medial temporal lobes, anterior thalamus, hypothalamic floor especially mammillary bodies); diffuse white matter atrophy, thinned corpus callosum; ventricular enlargement; septum pellucidum abnormalities (cavum, perforation, fenestration); pallor of locus coeruleus, substantia nigra.

The investigators[21] noted a predilection of p-*tau* pathology in the regions of dorsolateral frontal cortex, superior temporal cortex, entorhinal cortex, amygdala and locus coeruleus, with the youngest cases and lowest stage brains favoring p-*tau* depositions in dorsolateral frontal cortex and locus coeruleus. The investigators[21] also recommended further study of clinical expression correlation with CTE neuropathological staging, including risk factors enhancing susceptibility and disease progression.

These 2 studies outlined general paradigms of p-*tau* deposition in CTE throughout the human brain; however, much remains to be understood. For example, the amount and distribution of detectable p-*tau* accumulation in postmortem brain tissue samples, often seemingly cannot fully explain patient signs and symptoms, especially in low-stage cases (I/II) with limited p-*tau* pathology. In the 2 McKee staging papers, data showed patients with stage I CTE suffered from headache (70%), loss of attention (67%), executive function problems (70%), episodic memory difficulties (70%), depression (80%), and aggressive/explosive behaviors (55%).[9,21] Although a few patients displayed no symptoms, 15 patients (27.3%) had clinical dementia. Even at this early stage, a subset of patient brains showed neuropathology indicating comorbid neurodegenerative disease, such as Alzheimer disease, which may have at least partly contributed to individual patient clinical expression. The study design could not fully account for additional variables possibly contributing to clinical features, such as substance abuse. Clinical correlation becomes more muddled as deposition of p-*tau* increases in higher CTE stages. Other potential, yet largely unstudied, contributors to symptom expression include neuroinflammation, astrocytosis, and vascular abnormalities. Also, in all 4 stages, axonal abnormalities were noted, which may partially account for symptoms in affected patients and concomitantly as a source for pathologic p-*tau*.

Recent discoveries also raise questions about the uniqueness of the consensus pathognomonic lesion for CTE, especially as attributable solely to repetitive mild TBIs. Published before the consensus meeting, one neuropathology study revealed NFTs and glial cells with p-*tau* immunoreactivity, both situated in cortical sulcal depths, in postmortem brain tissues from long-term survivors of single moderate to severe TBI.[22] In addition, we studied the postmortem brains of 5 elderly patients with schizophrenia with histories of surgical leucotomies (severing axons bilaterally in prefrontal cortices) at least 40 years before death, as a human model of single, severe, and chronic axonal injury without external impact.[23] We discovered NFTs, astrocytic tangles, and p-*tau* immunoreactive neurites encompassing blood vessels in sulcal depths in irregular cortical spatial patterns in gray matter adjacent to the leucotomy sites. These findings suggest that chronic white matter axonal damage contributes to development of the p-*tau* pathognomonic signature of CTE, affecting cortical sulcal depths in close proximity. Findings fitting the proposed pathognomonic CTE lesion have also been noted in brain examinations of patients with head injury/substance abuse and neurodegenerative diseases including amyotrophic lateral sclerosis and multiple system atrophy.[8] Thus, the current nascent neuropathological definition for CTE diagnosis may represent brain injury from different circumstances, both traumatic and nontraumatic, which possibly share the commonality of axonal injury.

NEUROANATOMIC OVERLAP OF POSTTRAUMATIC STRESS DISORDER AND CHRONIC TRAUMATIC ENCEPHALOPATHY

In the past few decades of PTSD research, functional neuroimaging and animal studies have revealed identifiable, biological abnormalities in the brain, which can overlap with neuroanatomic sites associated with CTE. Pathophysiological dysfunction within specific neurocircuits presumably underlies symptoms of PTSD, such as fear learning, threat detection, contextual processing, and emotion regulation, often highlighting the amygdala and its reciprocal connections to other regions of the brain.[24–26] Briefly, amygdala hyperactivation may exaggerate fear learning, compounded with anterior cingulate and insular cortical hyperactivities inflating threat detection.[25,26] Hypo-responsiveness of ventromedial prefrontal (orbitofrontal) cortex possibly translates to decreased inhibitory output to the amygdala, which might additionally impair the coping function of fear extinction.[25] Moreover, patients with PTSD can display deficits in processing context (internal and external factors during a specific event affecting perception and memory, including fear regulation), which associates with connections among the hippocampus, ventromedial prefrontal cortex, amygdala, anterior cingulate cortex, and anterior insular cortex.[25,27] Patients with PTSD also often suffer from emotion dysregulation.[25,26] The ability to control and modulate emotions depends on several effective neurocircuits, especially in executive function, which commonly share the activation of dorsolateral prefrontal cortex.[24] Thus, both PTSD and CTE show evidence of compromise in amygdala, hippocampus, ventromedial prefrontal cortex, dorsolateral prefrontal cortex, anterior cingulate cortex, anterior insular cortex, and hypothalamus. Because the pathophysiology between head injury and CTE onset remains essentially unknown, the larger implication of this simple analysis is that physical damage from the head injury itself, in addition to physiologic reactions to the insult, may alter function of particularly vulnerable circuits.[28] It is therefore possible that an unknown percentage of patients diagnosed with PTSD potentially harbor uncharacterized lesions from TBI contributing to symptoms. In short, research studies of both PTSD and CTE imply dysfunction in overlapping neuroanatomic sites, which may translate into shared clinical symptoms in both medical conditions.

POTENTIAL MECHANISMS FOR *TAU* DEPOSITION IN CHRONIC TRAUMATIC ENCEPHALOPATHY

TBIs commonly produce axonal injury, a prominent factor often contributing to symptomatology in all injury severities (mild to severe) and concomitantly a potential source of p-*tau*.[29–31] Impact TBI is classically associated with diffuse axonal injury, with damage ranging from white matter of the cerebral hemispheres to the upper brainstem and cerebellum in more severe cases.[29,32] With mechanical disruption of the axonal cytoskeleton, proteins attached to microtubules accumulate at the site of damage.[31] As *tau* normally binds axonal microtubules, with damage *tau* can dissociate from microtubules, become hyperphosphorylated and likewise accumulate with the other proteins in axonal varicosities and bulbs. In both acute and remote TBI cases, immunoreactivity experiments with human brain tissues from surgical and postmortem patients revealed p-*tau* in damaged axons within white matter, as well as neurons and astrocytes within the human cerebral cortex.[9,33,34] Similarly, our research on leucotomized brains showed p-*tau* immunoreactivity in the cerebral cortex near axonal damage sites.[23] In another recent study of CTE cases, the investigators also reported an association between cortical sulci with high p-*tau* pathology and underlying white matter with axonal microstructural disruption.[35] Because traumatic axonal damage can persist for years, the impaired axons may provide a segue for p-*tau* to encroach the extracellular space insidiously over time.

In addition to p-*tau* accumulations after axonal injury, another biological phenomenon potentially affects brain protein aggregate formation after TBI, that is, prion-like dissemination. This hypothesis stems from the discovery of prions, which underlies the pathophysiology of Creutzfeldt-Jakob disease.[36] Briefly, with a genetic, sporadic, or transmissible initiation event, the endogenous human prion protein (PrP^C) changes conformation to the alternative isoform (PrP^{SC}), which can form aggregates, resist degradation and lead to neuronal toxicity and death.[37] By unclear mechanisms, PrP[SC] converts endogenous PrP[C] proteins to its toxic template isoform, propagating this deleterious conformational change through cellular networks (local proximity or synaptic neurocircuits), with consequent neurodegeneration and associated symptom expression. Likewise, multiple in vitro and in vivo studies showed uptake and propagation of *tau* prions in cell culture and human *tau* transgenic mouse brains, respectively, after inoculation with *tau* prion templates.[38–40] Specific to CTE, a recent cell culture study demonstrated that mammalian HEK293 T cells infected with *tau* proteins from human CTE postmortem brain extracts resulted in de novo *tau* prions in neighboring cells.[41] Last, in early CTE stages, postmortem human brains showed NFTs, astrocytic tangles, and p-*tau* neurites confined to the cortical sulcal depth.[9,21] In higher stages, neurons, astrocytes, and neurites of the 2 adjacent gyri also displayed p-*tau* immunoreactivity, in continuity with the original pathognomonic lesion at the cortical sulcal depth, which suggests spread within local cell networks. As with several tauopathies, however, *tau* prion theory does not fully explain the expansion of p-*tau* to other neuroanatomic sites (without apparent cellular network connectivity), inferring alternative biological mechanisms. Hence, the possibility exists that neurons and astrocytes in the human brain uptake extracellular p-*tau* formed after axonal injury and then propagate the conformational change through cellular networks.

One possible explanation for the pathognomonic p-*tau* accumulation pattern in CTE lies in interstitial solute clearance pathways in the human brain through local diffusion and fluid bulk flow, a process first proposed approximately 100 years ago with recent scientific breakthroughs. Unlike other physiologic systems of the human body, the brain lacks characteristic lymphatic vessels to provide protein and fluid homeostasis.[42] Rather, the human brain uses the glymphatic pathway, termed for its dependence on glial cells to function as the surrogate lymphatic system. In contemporary experiments involving rodents, data showed that cerebrospinal fluid (CSF) in the subarachnoid space influxes through periarterial spaces and exits through the aquaporin 4 channels of astrocytic endfeet into brain parenchyma. CSF then mixes with interstitial fluid (ISF) to flow through the interstitial space clearing macromolecules, including neurodegenerative proteins, and finally passes through aquaporin 4 channels of astrocytic endfeet around perivenous spaces to efflux from brain parenchyma.[42,43] In support of the hypothesis that CSF/ISF are essential components in a surrogate lymphatic system for the brain, 2 recent articles[44,45] provided evidence that CSF in mouse and human brain, with its soluble and cellular contents, flows into newly discovered lymphatic vessels in meninges lining dural sinuses that drain into cervical lymph nodes, in addition to other local lymphatic vessels of nasal mucosa, cranial nerve sheaths, and particular arteries and veins exiting the cranium. CSF also filtrates through arachnoid granulations to the dural venous sinuses, representing the only known CSF egress site draining directly into the bloodstream.[46] Furthermore, a seminal mouse study showed this CSF/ISF flushing process occurs most robustly during sleep, as the brains cleared β-amyloid proteins approximately two-fold faster than awake mice.[43] These study results infer the biological necessity of a functional glymphatic system, especially during sleep, to clear neurodegenerative proteins from the brain.

Other studies provide evidence that the glymphatic system specifically clears *tau* from the brain, and accordingly, malfunction of this system may promote p-*tau* accumulation after TBI with axonal injury. For instance, the investigators[47] of another contemporary mouse model article showed impaired function of the glymphatic system after TBI, with prominent reactive astrogliosis and glial scar formation, loss of perivascular aquaporin 4 polarization, axonal damage, and diminished interstitial *tau* clearance through perivascular pathways with accompanying p-*tau* increase in the brain. In the aquaporin 4 knockout mice subject to TBI, the brains showed profoundly impaired glymphatic clearance and higher levels of p-*tau*, in comparison to the brains from wild-type mice with TBI. Furthermore, the brains of the aquaporin 4 knockout mice with TBI displayed intense p-*tau* immunoreactivity in neuronal soma and surrounding neurites in immunohistochemistry experiments, suggesting higher levels of p-*tau* in the brain after TBI increases the likelihood of its detectable uptake in neighboring cells, including neurons. Based on these data, the investigators[47] proposed that prolonged impairment of perivascular clearance in the human brain after TBI potentially results in chronic pathologic accumulation of p-*tau*, leading to NFT and astrocytic tangle formation.

In the human brain with CTE, perivascular astrocytes in the neocortex display p-*tau* immunoreactivity, consistent with clearance data in rodents. Furthermore, considered a biomarker for axonal injury, total *tau* levels in humans increase in CSF and blood serum after TBI, including contact sports athletes shortly after mild TBIs.[48,49] Nonetheless, human brains with CTE show p-*tau* immunoreactivity in astrocytes, as well as neurons and neurites, specifically at cortical sulcal depths. Given most experiments involve rodents with lissencephalic brain structures, specific mechanisms of clearance within the human brain, particularly its relation to sulcal depths, remain poorly understood. For humans, the sulcal depth may serve as a site for *tau* clearance after axonal damage, whether by CSF/ISF flow patterns, cellular uptake or other mechanisms. In addition, TBI may cause alteration in astrocytic function with tissue damage. Pointedly, from sufficient physical head impact, mechanical stress can concentrate at the geometric inflection point of a sulcal depth.[22] As such, astrocytes in the damaged sulcus may alter cell programming from normal function to physiologic tissue repair, including change in aquaporin 4 localization (similar to mouse brain). If true, *tau* clearance pathways may be compromised at that site, with potential exacerbation of p-*tau* accumulation from underlying axonal injury leaking *tau* into the extracellular space. The mouse studies showed that increased *tau* concentration due to compromised glymphatic pathways resulted in neuronal as well as astrocytic uptake, inferring that concentration thresholds may account for the presence of NFTs at sulcal depths in CTE. Finally, differences in injury sites within the brain (sulcal depth, axonal injury) among individual patients may explain the apparent irregularity of the p-*tau* cortical spatial pattern observed years later at autopsy.

SUMMARY

Similar to other tauopathies, CTE diagnosis can be rendered at only autopsy. The final diagnosis represents one time point in the life of an individual patient, and requires consideration of available clinical history in conjunction with macroscopic examination and primarily p-*tau* accumulation patterns in the analysis of the postmortem brain. The continuum of pathophysiology from initial head injury to the development of CTE, however, is poorly understood. The initiating event of TBI can cause axonal injury, which may provide a continual source of *tau* to the extracellular environment. Current data pointing to the glymphatic pathway for clearance of fluids and proteins may explain the pathognomonic p-*tau* signature pattern of CTE, in addition to local neuron and astrocyte uptake of extracellular p-*tau* from damaged axons. Once in the intracellular compartment, p-*tau* potentially generates conformational changes in endogenous *tau*, which then propagates within cellular networks in a prion-like process at unknown rates. Because axonal injury can persist for years, the possibility exists that the balance between *tau* clearance pathways and potential neurodegenerative processes shifts to favor p-*tau* accumulation as clearance efficiency decreases with aging. This hypothetical, emergent imbalance perhaps partly explains the reported latency between initial TBI events and symptom expression in many patients with CTE.

In conclusion, clinicians still rely on nonspecific historical symptoms for diagnosis of PTSD, mild TBI, and CTE. The pathophysiology following TBI, and possibly leading to CTE, can alter function in vulnerable circuitry, which may contribute to deleterious clinical manifestations, potentially including symptoms of classic psychiatric diagnoses such as PTSD. The major limitation for all 3 diagnoses is the substantially unknown biology underpinning clinical expression, with the complication of probable heterogeneity in causality. Development of reliable neuroimaging and additional in vivo biomarkers for PTSD, TBI, CTE, and other TBI-related clinical entities, validated particularly with clinicopathologic correlation analysis, will allow for improved understanding of pathophysiological processes, ultimately leading to more effective and precise diagnostics, prognostics, and therapy.

CASE REPORT
History

A man in his 70s died in an assisted living facility. In his youth, he played American football throughout high school and college, and rugby after college until his mid-30s. He incurred many head injuries, which were "too numerous to count" according to family. One notable incident happened in his mid-20s when he suffered a knee blow to the head while playing rugby, which required hospitalization. His personality changed following this particular injury, and he was "never the same." In his adult life, he had several professions (real estate, accounting, education, coaching, painting). In his 40s, he developed mood disorder symptoms and was diagnosed with bipolar disorder. He married and divorced 3 times; the last divorce occurred in his 50s, and mainly for financial reasons. In his 60s, he developed progressive cognitive decline, including executive dysfunction and short-term memory loss. As time passed, he became less capable of performing activities of daily living. He also showed motor abnormalities. Ultimately, he moved to the dementia unit of an assisted living facility, where he lived for 3 years until his death.

Neuropathological Examination

The brain weight was slightly lower than expected, and gross examination revealed mild global atrophy, predominantly in the frontal and temporal lobes. The lateral and third ventricles showed enlargement; the third ventricles were disproportionately dilated with atrophy of the thalamus, hypothalamus, and mammillary bodies. The septum pellucidum displayed fenestrations (see **Fig. 2**A). The substantia nigra and locus coeruleus were pale. Microscopic and immunohistochemical examination of neocortex revealed abnormal aggregates of hyperphosphorylated *tau* (p-*tau*) in neurons (NFTs), astrocytes, and cell processes around small blood vessels (see **Fig. 2**D), preferentially in sulcal depths (see **Fig. 2**B). These aggregates formed individual foci within multiple lobes. In addition, the neocortex displayed numerous NFTs predominantly in superficial layers II-III, most pronounced in the frontal and temporal regions (see **Fig. 2**C). The thalamus, mammillary bodies, nucleus basalis of Meynert, substantia nigra, and locus coeruleus also showed neurofibrillary degeneration. Finally, the hippocampus contained NFTs, with a predilection for the second segment of the cornu ammonis (CA2). Immunohistochemical analyses for β-amyloid and α-synuclein revealed no significant burden.

Final Diagnosis

Chronic traumatic encephalopathy, McKee CTE Stage III.

ACKNOWLEDGMENTS

The authors thank Sofia Echelmeyer for her artistry in the illustrations. Funding,in part, was provided by the Defense Health Agency, U.S. Department of Defense.

DISCLOSURE

The opinions expressed herein are those of the authors and are not necessarily representative of those of the Uniformed Services University of the Health Sciences, the Department of Defense, or the US Army, Navy, or Air Force.

REFERENCES

1. Martland HS. Punch drunk. JAMA 1928;91(15):1103–7.
2. Critchley M. Punch-drunk syndromes: the chronic traumatic encephalopathy of boxers. Hommage a Clovis Vincent. Paris: Maloine; 1949.
3. Critchley M. Medical aspects of boxing, particularly from a neurological standpoint. Br Med J 1957;1(5015):357–62.
4. Brandenburg W, Hallervorden J. Dementia pugilistica with anatomical findings. Virchows Arch Pathol Anat Physiol Klin Med 1954;325:680–709.
5. Roberts AH. Brain damage in boxers: a study of the prevalence of traumatic encephalopathy among ex-professional boxers. London: Pitman Medical and Scientific Publishing; 1969.
6. McKee AC, Cairns NJ, Dickson DW, et al. The first NINDS/NIBIB consensus meeting to define neuropathological criteria for the diagnosis of chronic traumatic encephalopathy. Acta Neuropathol 2016;131(1):75–86.
7. Shively S, Scher AI, Perl DP, et al. Dementia resulting from traumatic brain injury: what is the pathology? Arch Neurol 2012;69(10):1245–51.
8. Iverson GL, Gardner AJ, Shultz SR, et al. Chronic traumatic encephalopathy neuropathology might not be inexorably progressive or unique to repetitive neurotrauma. Brain 2019;142(12):3672–93.
9. McKee AC, Stein TD, Nowinski CJ, et al. The spectrum of disease in chronic traumatic encephalopathy. Brain 2013;136(Pt 1):43–64.
10. Montenigro PH, Baugh CM, Daneshvar DH, et al. Clinical subtypes of chronic traumatic encephalopathy: literature review and proposed research diagnostic criteria for traumatic encephalopathy syndrome. Alzheimers Res Ther 2014; 6(5):68.
11. American Psychiatric Association. Diagnostic and statistical manual of mental disorders. 5th edition. Washington, DC: American Psychiatric Association; 2013.
12. Desmarais P, Weidman D, Wassef A, et al. The interplay between post-traumatic stress disorder and dementia: a systematic review. Am J Geriatr Psychiatry 2020; 28(1):48–60.
13. Günak MM, Billings J, Carratu E, et al. Post-traumatic stress disorder as a risk factor for dementia: systematic review and meta-analysis. Br J Psychiatry 2020; 217:600–8.
14. Bonanni L, Franciotti R, Martinotti G, et al. Post traumatic stress disorder heralding the onset of semantic frontotemporal dementia. J Alzheimers Dis 2018;63(1): 203–15.

15. Crary JF, Trojanowski JQ, Schneider JA, et al. Primary age-related tauopathy (PART): a common pathology associated with human aging. Acta Neuropathol 2014;128(6):755–66.
16. Tsartsalis S, Xekardaki A, Hof PR, et al. Early Alzheimer-type lesions in cognitively normal subjects. Neurobiol Aging 2018;62:34–44.
17. Braak H, Del Tredici K. The pathological process underlying Alzheimer's disease in individuals under thirty. Acta Neuropathol 2011;121(2):171–81.
18. Braak H, Thal DR, Ghebremedhin E, et al. Stages of the pathologic process in Alzheimer disease: age categories from 1 to 100 years. J Neuropathol Exp Neurol 2011;70(11):960–9.
19. Corsellis JA, Bruton CJ, Freeman-Browne D. The aftermath of boxing. Psychol Med 1973;3(3):270–303.
20. Hof PR, Bouras C, Buée L, et al. Differential distribution of neurofibrillary tangles in the cerebral cortex of dementia pugilistica and Alzheimer's disease cases. Acta Neuropathol 1992;85(1):23–30.
21. Alosco ML, Cherry JD, Huber BR, et al. Characterizing tau deposition in chronic traumatic encephalopathy (CTE): utility of the McKee CTE staging scheme. Acta Neuropathol 2020;140(4):495–512.
22. Johnson VE, Stewart W, Smith DH. Widespread τ and amyloid-β pathology many years after a single traumatic brain injury in humans. *Brain Pathol* 2012;22(2): 142–9.
23. Shively SB, Edgerton SL, Iacono D, et al. Localized cortical chronic traumatic encephalopathy pathology after single, severe axonal injury in human brain. Acta Neuropathol 2017;133(3):353–66.
24. Stahl SM. Stahl's essential psychopharmacology: neuroscientific basis and practical applications. 3rd edition. New York, NY: Cambridge University Press; 2008.
25. Sheynin J, Liberzon I. Circuit dysregulation and circuit-based treatments in posttraumatic stress disorder. Neurosci Lett 2017;649:133–8.
26. Shalev A, Liberzon I, Marmar C. Post-traumatic stress disorder. N Engl J Med 2017;376(25):2459–69.
27. Craig AD. How do you feel–now? The anterior insula and human awareness. Nat Rev Neurosci 2009;10(1):59–70.
28. Stein MB, McAllister TW. Exploring the convergence of posttraumatic stress disorder and mild traumatic brain injury. Am J Psychiatry 2009;166(7):768–76.
29. Strich SJ. Diffuse degeneration of the cerebral white matter in severe dementia following head injury. J Neurol Neurosurg Psychiatry 1956;19(3):163–85.
30. Oppenheimer DR. Microscopic lesions in the brain following head injury. J Neurol Neurosurg Psychiatry 1968;31(4):299–306.
31. Johnson VE, Stewart W, Smith DH. Axonal pathology in traumatic brain injury. Exp Neurol 2013;246:35–43.
32. Adams JH, Graham DI, Murray LS, et al. Diffuse axonal injury due to nonmissile head injury in humans: an analysis of 45 cases. Ann Neurol 1982;12:557–63.
33. Ikonomovic MD, Uryu K, Abrahamson EE, et al. Alzheimer's pathology in human temporal cortex surgically excised after severe brain injury. Exp Neurol 2004; 190(1):192–203.
34. Uryu K, Chen XH, Martinez D, et al. Multiple proteins implicated in neurodegenerative diseases accumulate in axons after brain trauma in humans. Exp Neurol 2007;208(2):185–92.
35. Holleran L, Kim JH, Gangolli M, et al. Axonal disruption in white matter underlying cortical sulcus tau pathology in chronic traumatic encephalopathy. Acta Neuropathol 2017;133(3):367–80.

36. Prusiner SB. Cell biology. A unifying role for prions in neurodegenerative diseases. Science 2012;336(6088):1511–3.
37. Venneti S. Prion diseases. Clin Lab Med 2010;30(1):293–309.
38. Clavaguera F, Bolmont T, Crowther RA, et al. Transmission and spreading of tauopathy in transgenic mouse brain. Nat Cell Biol 2009;11(7):909–13.
39. Frost B, Jacks RL, Diamond MI. Propagation of tau misfolding from the outside to the inside of a cell. J Biol Chem 2009;284(19):12845–52.
40. Sanders DW, Kaufman SK, DeVos SL, et al. Distinct tau prion strains propagate in cells and mice and define different tauopathies. Neuron 2014;82(6):1271–88.
41. Woerman AL, Aoyagi A, Patel S, et al. Tau prions from Alzheimer's disease and chronic traumatic encephalopathy patients propagate in cultured cells. Proc Natl Acad Sci U S A 2016;113(50):E8187–96.
42. Nedergaard M. Garbage truck of the brain. Science 2013;340(6140):1529–30.
43. Xie L, Kang H, Xu Q, et al. Sleep drives metabolite clearance from the adult brain. Science 2013;342(6156):373–7.
44. Aspelund A, Antila S, Proulx ST, et al. A dural lymphatic vascular system that drains brain interstitial fluid and macromolecules. J Exp Med 2015;212(7):991–9.
45. Louveau A, Smirnov I, Keyes TJ, et al. Structural and functional features of central nervous system lymphatic vessels. Nature 2015;523(7560):337–41.
46. Rasmussen MK, Mestre H, Nedergaard M. The glymphatic pathway in neurological disorders. Lancet Neurol 2018;17(11):1016–24.
47. Iliff JJ, Chen MJ, Plog BA, et al. Impairment of glymphatic pathway function promotes tau pathology after traumatic brain injury. J Neurosci 2014;34(49):16180–93.
48. Neselius S, Brisby H, Theodorsson A, et al. CSF-biomarkers in Olympic boxing: diagnosis and effects of repetitive head trauma. PLoS One 2012;7(4):e33606.
49. Shahim P, Tegner Y, Wilson DH, et al. Blood biomarkers for brain injury in concussed professional ice hockey players. JAMA Neurol 2014;71(6):684–92.

Neurobehavior and Mild Traumatic Brain Injury

Megan E. Solberg, MA[a], Silvana Riggio, MD[b,c,d],*

KEYWORDS

- Traumatic brain injury • Postconcussive syndrome • Neuropsychiatric disorders
- Depression • Cognition • Sleep disorders

KEY POINTS

- Up to 15% of patients with a mild traumatic brain injury experience neurobehavioral sequelae (somatic and neuropsychiatric complaints) at 1 year after injury.
- Nontraumatic brain injuries may have neurobehavioral sequelae presentations similar to those related to mild traumatic brain injury, emphasizing the importance of the differential diagnosis in approaching these patients.
- Impairment of attention and balance are hallmark neurobehavioral sequelae findings in the acute phase after a mild traumatic brain injury; headache is the most common somatic complaint.
- A number of risk factors, including premorbid mental illness and poor social support, have been related to the development of neurobehavioral sequelae.
- The management of neurobehavioral sequelae should focus on sleep hygiene, pain management, medication use and abuse, and other possible contributing factors.

INTRODUCTION

A traumatic brain injury (TBI) is often followed by neurobehavioral sequelae (NBS), which may include neuropsychiatric symptoms and/or somatic symptoms (**Box 1**). Much of the literature focuses on the sequelae from mild TBI (mTBI), which includes concussion, hence the term postconcussive symptoms or disorders. Furthermore, the majority of the recent literature focuses primarily on concussion in sports and

a Department of Counseling Psychology, Morgridge College of Education, University of Denver, 1999 East Evans Avenue, Denver, CO 80208, USA; b Department of Psychiatry, Mount Sinai School of Medicine, One Gustave L. Levy Place, Box 1230, New York, NY 10029, USA; c Department of Neurology, Mount Sinai School of Medicine, One Gustave L. Levy Place, Box 1230, New York, NY 10029, USA; d Department of Psychiatry, James J. Peters VAMC, 130 West Kingsbridge Road, Bronx, NY, USA
* Corresponding author. Department of Psychiatry, Icahn School of Medicine at Mount Sinai, 1425 Madison Avenue, New York, NY 10029.
E-mail address: silvana.riggio@mountsinai.org

Psychiatr Clin N Am 44 (2021) 459–468
https://doi.org/10.1016/j.psc.2021.04.004
0193-953X/21/© 2021 Elsevier Inc. All rights reserved.

Abbreviations	
mTBI	Mild traumatic brain injury
NBS	Neurobehavioral sequelae
TBI	Traumatic brain injury

caution should be exercised to avoid extrapolating this literature to the general population.

This article explores the NBS that may occur after a mTBI with a focus on the interface of NBS with other conditions; it provides a framework for developing a diagnostic and management strategy. The strategy must consider both acute and long-term recovery goals. Shared decision-making with a patient and early psychotherapeutic interventions (eg, supportive, family, group, cognitive behavioral therapies) are first-line strategies that may decrease symptom progression.[1] Despite the importance of pharmacotherapy in select cases, the benefit of medication needs to be weighed against its potential side effects that may interfere with function and recovery.

INCIDENCE

Up to 70% of patients with mTBI report some degree of NBS in the acute phase after injury. Indeed, normalizing the potential for developing symptoms is an important part of postdischarge planning in the acute phase of mTBI management.[2] Cognitive deficits are common in the acute stage, but most studies indicate that complete recovery is the norm for mTBI, generally within days to weeks and definitely within 3 to 12 months.[3] However, up to 15% of patients with mTBI report NBS beyond 3 months, which may contribute to long-term social and occupational difficulties. When this occurs, clinicians should look for contributing factors, including preexisting psychosocial variables.

Several variables have been identified that impact the evolution or resolution of NBS symptoms and complicate outcome prognostication. Symptoms can vary, depending on the localization and lateralization of the injury, extent of the injury, medical and psychiatric comorbidities, and psychosocial factors present, both before and after the injury. Moreover, individual coping mechanisms as well as social and economic support factors play a role in recovery.[4]

Box 1
NBS of TBI

Neuropsychiatric
• Cognitive: Deficits in attention, memory, and executive function
• Behavioral/psychiatric: Mood symptoms, aggression, irritability, poor impulse control, anhedonia, and apathy

Somatic
• Headaches
• Gait disturbance, dizziness, and vertigo
• Sleep disturbance
• Fatigue
• Seizures
• Visual disturbances
• Others

*Behavioral changes can be primarily due the injury and/or an exacerbation of predisposition of an underlying condition.

CLINICAL APPROACH

The evaluation of patients with a mTBI presenting with neurobehavioral complaints requires a systematic history and physical examination with a careful assessment of the complaints and contextualization of the injury, premorbid health, and postinjury circumstances. The evaluation should explore and characterize the presence of somatic symptoms including headaches, gait disturbance, dizziness, sleep disturbances, fatigue, seizures; and should explore neuropsychiatric symptoms including cognitive impairment, behavioral changes, and exacerbation of primary psychiatric disorders.

Clinical presentations are often complex to assess in the patient with mTBI and can overlap with psychiatric, neurologic, and or medical disorders, see **Fig. 1**. For example, post-traumatic seizures may complicate the presentation and diagnosis of post-TBI patients with suspected NBS. Specifically, seizures of frontal lobe origin can be associated with bizarre behavioral manifestations and repetitive motor activity, which risk being mistaken for a psychiatric presentation.[5]

Before anchoring on a diagnosis, a thorough physical examination is needed to ensure that a physical cause is not in play. For example, a subtle injury related to a 4th or 6th cranial nerve injury can contribute to headaches and difficulty concentrating or sustaining attention. After completion of the physical, neurologic and psychiatric evaluation, the clinician can properly determine an indication for any supplementary diagnostic studies (eg, neuroimaging, neurophysiologic, and/or neuropsychological testing).

NEUROBEHAVIORAL SEQUELAE
Cognitive Disorders

Cognitive dysfunction is a defining feature of mTBI. In a systematic review of the literature by Carney and colleagues,[6] it was reported as one of the most prevalent findings associated with mTBI. Specifically, a deficit in attention as evidenced by increased reaction time, impaired verbal learning, and impaired memory were found to be prevalent features of mTBI. A key feature in understanding the cognitive assessment is the principle that to remember one needs to be able to pay attention. Identifying these

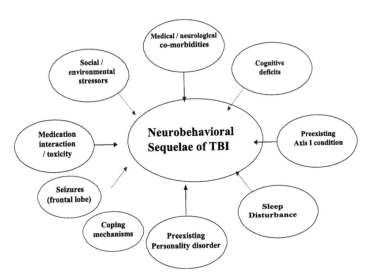

Fig. 1. Concomitant factors of NBS sequelae.

deficits and developing an effective intervention plan may be pivotal to the successful recovery of the patient.

Risk factors for persisting symptoms, in addition to structural injury, include female sex, advanced age, pain, and prior mood symptoms.[7] Neither loss of consciousness nor post-traumatic amnesia reliably stratifies those patients at greatest risk for cognitive deficits.[6]

In the acute phase (eg, on the sidelines), cognition is often assessed using a standardized evaluation form, such as the SCAT5. In the subacute and chronic periods, this evaluation may be performed using neuropsychologic testing tool, which can be either paper and pencil or computer based. A challenge to interpreting the findings of cognitive tests may be the lack of a baseline for comparison.

When cognitive impairment is identified, the clinician must then determine if the cause is due to the injury itself or due to some other confounding condition (eg, pain, medication, and/or preexisting comorbidities). Mild TBI–related deficits in attention and information processing may interfere with the performance of preinjury tasks. Patients often report difficulty sustaining attention, planning, switching parameters, organizing, or sequencing. These deficits may result in frustration and be expressed in the form of increased irritability, anxiety, apathy, or depression. Clinicians must determine if these symptoms are the result of the injury per se (ie, injury to the frontal lobe) or a manifestation of the frustration of not performing at their premorbid baseline.

The post-TBI evaluation of cognitive function must determine if performance problems are due to deficits in attention versus memory.[8] If attention is impaired, there is difficulty retaining information with an obvious impact on memory and thus performance. If a patient has an underlying affective disorder, attention can also be impaired owing to a lack of interest and/or distractibility. Therefore, the assessment of memory must be placed in the context of attention and other disorders that may interfere with performance.

The sports medicine literature on mTBI has reported that cognitive impairments are most severe immediately after the closed head injury and generally resolve within 2 to 3 months, and rarely lasting more than 3 months.[9,10]

Another important factor to consider when talking about cognition and TBI is the possible risk associated with repetitive concussions, cumulative head impact exposure, and the long-term effects of TBI, like the progressive cognitive decline associated with normal aging and or neurodegenerative disorders (eg, long-term risks for Chronic Traumatic Encephalopathy [CTE]). These issues are particularly important in the evaluation of athletes who are at risk for multiple concussions. However, to this day there is a lack of well-designed prospective studies, with consequent limitations in obtaining quality data. Little is known regarding the incidence of recurrent concussion or whether repetitive concussion or head impact exposure leads to cognitive impairment either directly or indirectly.

Behavioral and Psychiatric Disorders

A behavioral complaint after a mTBI could be due to the injury, might have been present before the injury, or there may have been a predisposition not manifested until the injury. Although an area of intense research, the literature is not clear on whether mTBI in and of itself directly causes lasting behavioral disorders. For example, in a well-designed retrospective study by Voormolen and colleagues,[11] 1000 patients with mTBI were compared with 1000 patients without TBI; the results indicated that neurobehavioral symptoms are prominent in the general population and thus are not unique to TBI injury. Regardless, it is not uncommon for patients and/or their family and friends to comment that there is a change in behavior after an mTBI, although the change is often very difficult for them to qualify.

The family and the patient's history may be key to understanding the presenting complaint. A recent study found that high school athletes with mTBI were 5 times more likely to experience prolonged recovery if they had a family or personal psychiatric history, particularly for anxiety or bipolar disorder.[12] Weak defense mechanisms, poor social support, medications, and drug use can all complicate the presentation. Complex symptoms can also be impacted by an emotional response to the injury, its limitations, and the fear of disability (see **Fig. 1**).

Aggression

Aggression is reported more commonly after moderate and severe TBI than after mTBI. Risk factors for aggression after mTBI include frontal lobe injury, a premorbid affective disorder, personality disorder, and alcohol and/or substance use. Aggressive behavior in military personnel with mTBI has been identified as a precursor to depression and suicide risk, suggesting that clinical interventions targeting anger may inhibit the pathway to suicide risk in this group.[13]

Depression

Major depression is one of the most frequently reported NBS of TBI; the actual prevalence varies from study to study based on methodology, but has generally been reported to be significantly higher than the 17% incidence in the general population.[14–16] Most research to date is not prospective in nature and, thus, causation between mTBI and depression is still not well-understood, but this finding underscores the need to acknowledge that a risk exists.

The degree to which a premorbid psychiatric disorder increases the risk for NBS after mTBI is unclear, but studies indicate a positive correlation.[17,18] Risk factors for developing major depression after TBI fall into 2 categories: premorbid psychiatric pathology and low socioeconomic status. Roy and colleagues[17] found a significant association between decreased social functioning after TBI and new-onset depression after a first TBI in 103 subjects at 3, 6, and 12 months after the injury. No sex difference has been reported in mTBI studies.[18]

There is conflicting evidence linking mTBI and suicidality. In a retrospective study of 5034 patients, Silver and colleagues[19,20] reported that patients with mTBI with a loss of consciousness had a 4 times greater likelihood of attempted suicide than those without TBI (8% vs 2%). This risk of suicide attempt remained even after controlling for demographics, quality-of-life variables, alcohol abuse, and any comorbid psychiatric disorders. Conversely, in a systematic review of the literature, Hesdorffer and colleagues[20] found insufficient evidence linking mTBI and completed suicide.

Anxiety Disorders and Post-traumatic Stress Disorder

There is an association between mTBI and stress disorders, but as with other neurobehavioral symptoms discussed, the relationship is complex. Increased age, an avoidant coping style, and a history of post-traumatic stress disorder are potential risk factors for acute stress symptoms after TBI.[21] An awareness of this risk helps to guide the treatment plan, including return to baseline activities.

There is some evidence that mTBI may experience a higher rate of combined anxiety and depression symptoms as opposed to singular depression. Barker-Collo and colleagues[15] studied 877 patients with mTBI over 4 years and reported that depression without anxiety occurs less frequently than singular anxiety (3.7%–29.5%) and comorbid anxiety and depression (10.2%–20.7% over the first 12 months after TBI and 11.8% at 4 years after TBI). Regardless, this study and others establish an association but fall short of establishing a cause and effect of mTBI as the primary cause of anxiety, depression, or other mood disorders.

Along the same lines, acute stress disorder may predispose a patient with mTBI to develop post-traumatic stress disorder, but a cause-and-effect relationship is unclear. Because recall of a traumatic event is a contributing factor to developing post-traumatic stress disorder, it has been proposed that the loss of consciousness or post-traumatic amnesia seen in some mTBI cases may be protective against the development of post-traumatic stress disorder by inhibiting access to traumatic memories.[22,23]

The primary question is how patients can have post-traumatic stress disorder if they cannot re-experience the actual trauma via intrusive thoughts or nightmares. The proposed counterargument in the controversy is the theory that patients with TBI with post-traumatic amnesia for a traumatic event re-experience the trauma event through the imagination from secondhand accounts or the patient's own mind and that patients may also be able to re-experience fragments or islands of memory within the amnestic period, thus meeting the re-experiencing criterion of post-traumatic stress disorder.[24] The best available evidence on the relationship between TBI and post-traumatic stress disorder comes from a military study by Hoge and colleagues[25]; after adjusting for post-traumatic stress disorder and depression, they reported that mTBI was not significantly associated with post-traumatic stress disorder. The investigators postulated that post-traumatic stress disorder and depression are important mediators of the relationship between mTBI and physical health problems.

Substance-Related Disorders

Premorbid substance use has been found to be strongly associated with post-TBI drug use, and many studies have cited substance abuse as a risk factor for TBI rather than vice versa. A 30-year longitudinal study by Koponen and colleagues[26] showed that 71% of patients with TBI who were using drugs currently also did so before TBI.

SOMATIC SYMPTOMS

The somatic sequelae of TBI often complicate the neurobehavioral presentations, underscoring the importance of an integrated approach to evaluating these patients.

Headache

Headache is the most commonly reported somatic symptom after mTBI.[8] Post-TBI headaches are classified either as acute, beginning within 2 weeks of the injury and resolving within 2 months, or as chronic, beginning within 2 weeks and persisting for more than 8 weeks. A history of headaches increases the risk of having headaches after mTBI, although the majority resolve within 3 months.[27]

Post-mTBI headache commonly co-occurs with other NBS symptoms. Baandrup and Jensen[28] reported that 53% of patients had at least 1 other somatic complaint (eg, fatigability, sleep disturbance, dizziness, or alcohol intolerance), 49% had at least 1 cognitive complaint (eg, memory dysfunction or impaired concentration/attention), 26% had at least 1 psychiatric complaint (eg, irritability, aggressiveness, anxiety, depression, or emotional lability), 17% had all 3 types of complaints, and 17% had none.

Dizziness

Dizziness (inclusive of lightheadedness, disequilibrium, loss of balance, and vertigo) is the second most commonly reported somatic complaint after head injury, although most studies do not separate the vague complaint of dizziness from those of vertigo.[8] The pathophysiology of post-traumatic dizziness may be due to either injury to the central nervous system and or to the peripheral vestibular system. The etiology must be teased apart in the history and physical examination. Dizziness can have a major impact on overall well-being and may contribute to anxiety and other NBS. Anticholinergics (eg, meclizine) should be used judiciously, if at all, in treating patients with a complaint of dizziness; their sedative properties often make patients feel worse and may contribute to falls and injury.

Fatigue and Sleep Disturbance

Fatigue occurs in up to 70% of patients with mTBI and complicates the assessment of depression in these patients. Like other somatic symptoms, it typically improves within 3 months. It has been reported in up to 73% of patients after a TBI.[29] Post-TBI fatigue can be disabling and its etiology may be complex and multifactorial. Pain, sleep disorders, cognitive deficits, mood disorders, medical comorbidities, a lack of physical exercise, and medications are several of the contributing factors. The presence of fatigue can be associated with poorer social integration, a decreased level of productive activities, and a decreased overall quality of life. When fatigue persists, it may present a barrier to recovery.

A sleep disturbance is yet another frequently reported NBS. Studies on veterans who sustained an mTBI during deployment have indicated a significantly increased incidence of poor sleep quality compared with veterans without a history of mTBI, even when combat exposure and behavioral health issues were taken into consideration.[30] This study and others suggest that mTBI should be considered as a potential contributor to sleep disturbances. Key to managing sleep disorders is identifying the factors contributing to the presentation. Because sleep disturbances are known to contribute to neurocognitive and neurobehavioral deficits and increased recovery time after a TBI, early intervention may improve patient outcomes and reduce secondary effects of TBI.

Seizures

Owing to the high incidence of TBI to the frontal or temporal lobe, the focus of post-traumatic seizures is often in these areas. Seizures of a frontal lobe origin can be difficult to diagnose because they can present with a wide variety of clinical manifestations, frequently mimicking psychiatric disorders, yet can have a normal electroencephalogram.[5] The bizarreness of frontal lobe seizures, without associated tonic–clonic activity or loss of consciousness, results in the diagnosis frequently being overlooked. A key point is that when agitation, brief outbursts of rage and aggression, and/or new-onset bizarre behavior occur in association with a history of TBI, a detailed history and careful characterization of the events are warranted. If the episodes are periodic, stereotypic, and brief in duration with a variable postictal phase, then the possibility of a frontal lobe seizure should be entertained.

PUTTING IT ALL TOGETHER

Evaluating the NBS of mTBI requires a detailed understanding of a patient's neurologic, psychiatric, and primary illnesses both before and after the injury and include a careful assessment of potential contributory factors. At times, it can be difficult to differentiate NBS after mTBI from similar symptomatology secondary to a preexistent disorder. The literature reports a high incidence of both neurobehavioral and somatic complaints after a TBI, but caution must be used because many of these studies are underpowered, retrospective, or flawed by bias. In addition, many of the studies include patients of all TBI severities and include patients with prior psychiatric and substance abuse histories. Adding to the controversy surrounding mTBI and NBS are studies showing that patients with non–TBI-related injuries have an incidence of neurobehavioral complaints similar to those associated with TBI.[31,32]

A major question confronting mental health providers is how best to treat the patient with mTBI with mood symptoms; that is, how to prioritize psychotherapy and pharmacotherapeutic interventions. This goal can only be accomplished by performing a comprehensive medical and behavioral assessment. The evaluation must determine the relative contributions of central nervous system lesions, physical disabilities, and environmental stressors. There are inherent risks of pharmacotherapy, especially when a patient is cognitively compromised after a TBI. Antidepressants can interfere with cognitive function, especially with attention and memory, and can cause sleep disturbances.

Clinicians must be vigilant against premature closure when diagnosing a behavioral presentation as psychiatric. For example, patients with TBI with a depressed mood may have a major depressive disorder, but could also have an adjustment disorder with depressed mood, a lesion in the mesial frontal region, injury to the basal ganglia, or hypothyroidism. An adjustment disorder might not require pharmacotherapy, whereas a major depression disorder does; depression from a mesial frontal lesion would have questionable benefit from antidepressants. Depression from a basal ganglia lesion could potentially get worse with antidepressants owing to the possibility of secondary extrapyramidal symptoms with bradykinesia mimicking psychomotor retardation. Not only must the cause of the depression be determined, but also clinicians must remember the possibly that the depression may be an expression of an existing condition and not directly owing to the TBI. A key point is the need for clinicians to avoid bias and regularly reassess the patient's response to treatments; screening for suicidality is always indicated in that symptoms can fluctuate as well as an individual's ability to adapt to possible life changes after a TBI.

Cognitive deficits are hallmarks of mTBI and their recognition is fundamental to a successful management plan. The differential diagnosis of cognitive dysfunction (eg, deficits in attention) includes structural lesions, an underlying medical problem, a primary psychiatric disorder, or a drug side effect (in particular, compounds with high anticholinergic properties or antihistaminergic properties). Sleep disturbances and pain syndromes can also interfere with attention. Attention can be affected by a lesion in the orbitofrontal region, resulting in high distractibility, or a lesion in the dorsolateral region, resulting in an inability to switch mindset or multitask. Mood disorders and anxiety are yet additional factors to take into consideration because they too may impact attention.

The NBS from a TBI are common but fortunately resolve in the majority of patients in the weeks to months after injury. When they persist, a multidisciplinary team approach is often indicated. Family involvement is important to promote an understanding and support system needed for successful management. The literature on mTBI demonstrates that education alone can decrease the severity and duration of NBS, partially by normalizing the situation and providing the reassurance needed to promote recovery.[3]

REFERENCES

1. Roy D, Koliatsos V, Vaishnavi S, et al. Risk factors for new-onset depression after first-time traumatic brain injury. Psychosomatics 2018;59(1):47–57.

2. Ponsford J, Willmott C, Rothwell A. Impact of early intervention on outcome following mild head injury in adults. J Neurol Neurosurg Psych 2002;73:330–2.

3. Carroll LJ, Cassidy JD, Peloso PM, et al. Prognosis for mild traumatic brain injury: results of the WHO collaborating center task force on mild traumatic brain injury. J Rehabil Med 2004;(Suppl 43):84–105.

4. van der Naalt J, Timmerman M, de Koning M, et al. Early predictors of outcome after mild traumatic brain injury (UPFRONT): an observational cohort study. Lancet 2017;16:532–40.

5. Riggio S, Harner RN. Repetitive motor activity in frontal lobe epilepsy. In: Jasper H, Riggio S, Goldman-Rakic PS, editors. Epilepsy and the frontal anatomy of the frontal lobe. New York (NY): Raven Press; 1995. p. 153–66.

6. Carney N, Ghajar J, Jagoda A, et al. Executive summary of concussion guidelines Step I: systematic review of prevalent indicators. Neurosurg 2014;75:S1–2.

7. Meares S, Shores EA, Taylor AJ, et al. Mild traumatic brain injury does not predict acute postconcussion syndrome. J Neurol Neurosurg Psychiatry 2008;79:300.

8. Lumba-Brown A, Teramoto M, Bloom OJ, et al. Concussion guidelines step 2: evidence for subtype classification. Neurosurgery 2020;86(1):2–13.

9. McCrea M, Guskiewicz KM, Marshall SW, et al. Acute effects and recovery time following concussion in collegiate football players: the NCAA concussion study. J Am Med Assoc 2003;290:2556–63.

10. McAllister T, McCrea M. Long-term cognitive and neuropsychiatric consequences of repetitive concussion and head impact exposure. J Athl Train 2017; 52:309–17.

11. Voormolen DC, Cnossen MC, Polinder S, et al. Prevalence of post-concussion-like symptoms in the general population in Italy, The Netherlands and the United Kingdom. Brain Inj 2019;33(8):1078–86.

12. Legarreta AD, Brett BL, Solomon GS, et al. The role of family and personal psychiatric history in postconcussion syndrome following sport-related concussion: a story of compounding risk. J Neurosurg Pediat 2018;22:238–43.

13. Stanley IH, Joiner TE, Bryan CJ. Mild traumatic brain injury and suicide risk among a clinical sample of deployed military personnel: evidence for a serial mediation model of anger and depression. J Psychiatr Res 2017;84:161–8.

14. Bombardier CH, Fann JR, Dikmen SS, et al. Rates of major depressive disorder and clinical outcomes following traumatic brain injury. JAMA 2010;303:1938–45.

15. Barker-Collo S, Theadom A, Jones K, et al. Depression and anxiety across the first 4 years after mild traumatic brain injury: findings from a community-based study. Brain Inj 2018;32(13–14):1651–8.

16. Singh R, Mason S, Lecky F, et al. Comparison of early and late depression after TBI; (the SHEFBIT study). Brain Inj 2019;33(5):584–91.

17. Roy D, Peters ME, Everett A, et al. Loss of consciousness and altered mental state predicting depressive and post-concussive symptoms after mild traumatic brain injury. Brain Inj 2019;33(8):1064–9.

18. Barker-Collo S, Jones A, Jones K, et al. Prevalence, natural course and predictors of depression 1 year following traumatic brain injury from a population-based study in New Zealand. Brain Inj 2015;29(7–8):859–65.

19. Silver JM, Kramer R, Greenwald S, et al. The association between head injuries and psychiatric disorders: findings from the new haven NIMH epidemiologic catchment area study. Brain Inj 2001;15:935–45.

20. Hesdorffer D, Rauch S, Tamminga C. Long term psychiatric outcomes following traumatic brain injury: a review of the literature. J Head Trauma Rehabil 2009; 24:452–9.

21. Harvey AG, Bryant RA. Predictors of acute stress following mild traumatic brain injury. Brain Inj 1998;12:147–54.
22. Gil S, Caspi Y, Ben-Ari IZ, et al. Does memory of a traumatic event increase the risk of posttraumatic stress disorder in patients with traumatic brain injury? A prospective study. Am J Psychiatry 2005;162:963–9.
23. Turnbull SJ, Campbell EA, Swann IJ. Post-traumatic stress disorder symptoms following a head injury: does amnesia for the event influence the development of symptoms? Brain Inj 2001;15:775–85.
24. Bryant RA, Marosszeky JE, Crooks J, et al. Coping style and post-traumatic stress disorder following severe traumatic brain injury. Brain Inj 1999;14:175–80.
25. Hoge CW, McGurk D, Thomas JL, et al. Mild traumatic brain injury in soldiers returning from Iraq. N Engl J Med 2008;358:453–63.
26. Koponen S, Taiminen T, Portin R. Axis I and II psychiatric disorders after traumatic brain injury: a 30-year follow-up study. Am J Psychiatry 2002;159:1315–21.
27. Sufrinko A, Mc Allister, Deitrich J, et al. Family history of migraine associated with posttraumatic migraine symptoms following sports related concussion. J Head Trauma Rehabil 2018;131:17–24.
28. Baandrup L, Jensen R. Chronic post-traumatic headache—a clinical analysis in relation to the International Headache Classification 2nd Edition. Cephalgia 2005;25:132–8.
29. Cantor JB, Ashman T, Gordon W, et al. Fatigue after traumatic brain injury and its impact on participation and quality of life. J Head Trauma Rehabil 2008;23:41–51.
30. Rao V, Rollings P. Sleep disturbances following traumatic brain injury. Curr Treat Options Neurol 2002;4:77–87.
31. Iverson GL, McCracken LM. 'Postconcussive' symptoms in persons with chronic pain. Brain Inj 1997;11:783–90.
32. Hart RP, Martelli MF, Zasler ND. Chronic pain and neuropsychological functioning. Neuropsychol Rev 2000;10:131–49.

Psychosocial Aspects of Sport-Related Concussion in Youth

Aaron S. Jeckell, MD[a],*, R. Shea Fontana, DO[b]

KEYWORDS

- Sport concussion • Psychosocial factors • Concussion recovery

KEY POINTS

- Sport-related concussion (SRC) has the potential to affect an individual in several biological, psychological, and social ways.
- Media portrayal and public perception of SRC has the potential to affect recovery from injury and participation in youth sports.
- Our understanding of SRC has improved over the years, and current management guidelines reflect our evolving knowledge.
- Guidelines exist to help guide management and promote recovery from concussion in a way that takes psychological and social factors into account.

INTRODUCTION

Participation in youth sports and athletics has been a cornerstone of childhood development for generations. Ample evidence reinforces the value of physical activity starting at a young age with participation in team sport, as compared with individual sport, conferring additional psychosocial benefits. However, participation in any physical activity carries certain risk of injury. Chief among this is exposure to possible concussion or mild traumatic brain injury (mTBI). Sport-related concussion (SRC) has come into focus as having a tremendous impact in medical, academic, and social domains. While briefly addressing some of the biology and history of concussion, the authors explore the myriad of ways that SRC has affected the individual, family, and community on a psychosocial level.

[a] Department of Psychiatry and Behavioral Health, Vanderbilt University School of Medicine, 1500 21st Avenue South, Nashville, TN 37212, USA; [b] Department of Psychiatry and Behavioral Health, University of South Carolina School of Medicine – Greenville, Prisma Health – Upstate, 10 Patewood Drive, Suite 130, Greenville, SC 29615, USA
* Corresponding author.
E-mail address: Aaron.jeckell.md@gmail.com

Psychiatr Clin N Am 44 (2021) 469–480
https://doi.org/10.1016/j.psc.2021.04.013
0193-953X/21/© 2021 Elsevier Inc. All rights reserved.

A HISTORICAL PERSPECTIVE

As our understanding of concussion has evolved, so has the consideration surrounding the risks and benefits of participating in youth sport. In the early 1900s, concern over the morbidity and mortality associated with head injury in collegiate football mounted. Physicians at the time noted that football players and boxers who experienced multiple concussions had the potential to experience long-term disability. Some of the first descriptions relating to SRC were done in 1928 by Harrison Martland in his seminal work on boxers, "Punch Drunk."[1] The athletes in question experienced TBI of various severity levels. Some who experienced severe brain injury developed long-term neurologic and psychological impairment. The term *dementia pugilistica* was used to describe tremors, slowed movement, speech problems, and confusion seen in some of these fighters. This early conceptualization of concussion included a range of brain injuries and varies considerably from the more nuanced understanding we have today for SRC.

CURRENT SCOPE OF THE PROBLEM
Defining Concussion

The Concussion in Sport Group led by McCrory et al (2017) defines SRC as an mTBI induced by a biomechanical force that is transmitted to the brain. After a concussive injury, an individual likely experiences a rapid onset of short-lived neuropsychiatric symptoms that resolve spontaneously over days to weeks. Common symptoms associated with concussion include physical signs (loss of consciousness, dizziness), behavioral changes (depression, irritability, anxiety), cognitive impairment (amnesia, delayed reaction speed, inattention, poor concentration, memory disturbance), sleep disturbance, fatigue, and somatic symptoms (nausea, headache). Although SRC may cause biological and neurochemical changes on the microscopic level, symptoms represent a functional impairment rather than structural damage to the central nervous system or associated organ systems on a macroscopic level. Commonly used forms of neuroimaging (radiography, computed tomography, MRI) are expected to be negative (**Box 1**).[2]

On a cellular level, the impact that causes a concussion leads to a complex neurochemical cascade involving dysregulation of neurologic ions and neurotransmitters as well as increases in free radicals and other mediators of inflammation. As neurobiological processes take place to bring the neurochemistry back into equilibrium, the brain requires additional energy in the form of oxygen and glucose provided through vascular circulation. Another consequence of mTBI is a period of decreased cerebral blood flow, leading to a disparity in the amount of energy being provided to the brain relative to what it needs to restore homeostasis. This energy inequity is believed to be the cause of the functional impairments seen in SRC and other mTBI.[3,4]

Epidemiology of Concussion

Estimates suggest that 1.6 to 3.8 million Americans experience an SRC in the United States every year, including those who do not seek medical care.[5] Concussion is a type of injury that disproportionally affects youth and athlete populations.[6] TBI among youth athletes (0–19 years old) alone contributes 173,285 emergency department visits per year.[7]

Concussion in youth athletics has been increasing in the past several decades with a rate of 0.12/1000 athlete exposures (AE) in 1998 increasing to 0.49/1000 AE in 2008.[8] The authors have developed additional clarity regarding which sports place athletes at the highest risk for concussion, with rugby (4.18/1000 AE), ice hockey (1.2/1000 AE),

---

Box 1
Features of sport-related concussion

- SCR is caused by in impact somewhere on the body with the force being transmitted to the brain. An individual does not need to be hit on the head to experience a concussion.

- SRC typically results in the impairment of neuropsychiatric signs and symptoms that develop within minutes to hours and resolve over the course of days to weeks.

- Impairments are expected to resolve in a gradual and stepwise manner over the course of days to weeks.

- SRC may cause neuropathological and neurochemical changes, but gross neuroimaging is expected to be negative. Neuropsychiatric signs and symptoms represent a functional disturbance rather than response to structural injury.

- SRC can result in a range of signs and symptoms that include somatic symptoms, cognitive impairment, sleep disturbance, and emotional dysregulation.

- Most of the SRC do not result in loss of consciousness, which is not required to make a diagnosis of concussion.

- Resolution of symptoms typically follows a sequential course over the days to weeks. Most of the cases resolve within 30 days, with multiple factors having the potential to prolong recovery.

Data from McCrory P, Meeuwisse W, Dvorak J, et al. Consensus statement on concussion in sport-the 5th international conference on concussion in sport held in Berlin, October 2016. *Br J Sports Med.* 2017;51(11):838-847.

---

and American football (0.53/1000 AE) being the greatest contributors.[9] Whether the increase in youth SRC is due to an increase in the rate of injury or improved sophistication in detecting concussion remains unclear. Regardless, the rate of mTBI is high, and having an appropriate understanding of this type of injury is crucial for managing outcomes.

SOCIAL IMPACT OF CONCUSSION
Decline in Sport Participation

Along with developments in our understanding of SRC, a demographic shift in youth athletics has been occurring. Despite new rules and laws that enhance sport safety, certain youth sports are seeing a decrease in participation for the first time in decades. In the 2018 to 2019 season there were 7,937,491 student athletes participating in high school sports, a decline of 43,395 from the previous year. The most significant decreases were in football and basketball.[10] In 2018, tackle football participation was down 1.8% from the previous year, with a 5.8% drop in core participation (playing 26+ times a year).[11] Although the reasons for decreases in participation are multifactorial, risk of injury and concussion has been cited as a primary driving factor.[10]

Public Perception of Sport-Related Concussion

Surveys have demonstrated that parents have a high level of concern about their children being exposed to SRC; this is most significant in youth football followed by soccer.[12] Thirty-two percent of parents have expressed fear that their child will experience a concussion.[13] A quarter of all parents have considered removing their children from sports due to this concern.[12,13] A great deal of this anxiety is both precipitated and perpetuated by media representation of the mixed data surrounding SRC and high profile cases of professional athletes who have been affected by SRC.

Media Portrayal of Concussed Athletes

Media representation of concussed athletes has the potential to influence public perception of SRC.[14] In some cases, portrayal of SRC may precipitate fear and dread, whereas underreporting or misrepresenting the true nature of SRC could stall help-seeking practices. In some cases, athletes who play through injuries, including concussions, are viewed as being resilient or even heroic; this can perpetuate a narrative that athletes are expected to put their physical well-being at risk for the benefit of the team or their own personal performance. This portrayal may also underscore the severity of an injury such as SRC, leading young athletes to underestimate the risks associated with playing while injured or in recovery.

Media Representation of Medical Literature on Sport-Related Concussion

There are currently many gaps in the medical research examining short- and long-term consequences of SRC. For instance, several papers have established a link between early exposure to football and cognitive impairment later in life.[15–17] Other studies have failed to replicate these findings or been unable to establish a similar causal link.[18–22] There are mixed data regarding who is more likely to experience a prolonged recovery from concussion and why, and the medical community does not fully understand what factors may cause SRC in one individual but not in another.[23] The conflicting information and knowledge gaps have the potential to leave the public confused and uncertain about the validity of expert recommendations.

To compound this, media outlets have seized on research examining high-profile athletes with chronic traumatic encephalopathy (CTE) pathology.[24] An example of this is the work published by Mez and colleagues[25] In a convenience sample of individuals whose brains were donated to a CTE research group, 99% of National Football League (NFL) football players, 91% of college football players, and 21% of high school football players were found on autopsy to have neuropathology consistent with CTE. These findings sent shockwaves through popular media and nonmedical sources, and several professional athletes retired in response. However, this work was not without serious limitations that were not conveyed in the lay press. Media outlets ran stories suggesting that 99% of former NFL players have CTE.[26] Because this was a convenience sample, it does not provide an accurate representation of former NFL players. The brains in this study were donated for research, many due to concerns of neuropsychiatric findings that these individuals demonstrated while alive. This ascertainment bias can be significant, and there was no control group to compare rates of pathology with. The investigators of that paper even noted that, "…caution must be used in interpreting the high frequency of CTE in this sample, and estimates of prevalence cannot be concluded or implied from this sample."[25]

Ultimately, the percentage of current and former athletes who develop CTE is unknown, and our understanding of the links between participation in sport, SRC, and CTE remains unclear.[27,28] Nonetheless, it is reasonable to speculate that decreases in participation in youth sport and prominent worry over SRC have been fueled by media coverage of this injury.[29,30]

EVALUATING THE DECISION TO RETURN TO ACTIVITY
Return to Activity

SRC is expected to follow a gradual and stepwise resolution of symptoms.[2] Most of the SRC resolve relatively quickly (<10–14 days for adults, <4 weeks for youths).[2] Recovery from SRC is often facilitated by an initial period of 24 to 48 hours of physical and cognitive rest followed by careful adherence to gradual and regulated return-to-play (RTP) and return-to-learn (RTL) protocols[2] (**Table 1**). These protocols are designed to progressively reintegrate an individual into the academic and sport setting while mitigating and accounting for possible exacerbation of symptoms due to over-exertion. It is typical for student athletes to be expected to complete an RTL before engaging in an RTP. A multidisciplinary team consisting of the athlete, parents/guardians, academic personnel, coaches, trainers, and medical providers should be engaged during the rehabilitative process.[31] If concussion-related symptoms worsen or persist with activity, the individual should rest and return to the previous step. If these symptoms persist over a period of time that is longer than would be expected, referral to a clinician with expertise in the management of concussion is warranted.[32] In addition to the steps outlined in **Table 1**, Davis-Hayes and colleagues proposed both absolute and relative contraindications to return to sport[33] (**Table 2**).

The guidelines for returning to play post-SRC are specific to adult athletes and may differ to some degree depending on age, with adult and professional athletes typically progressing faster than youth and amateur athletes. At this time there are limited guidelines specific for youth athletes, although many providers advocate for a more conservative rehabilitation strategy due to the risk of injury in the developing brain.[34]

Over the last decade, the medical community has gained a new perspective in the treatment practices following SRC. Previously, a common treatment strategy advised strict and prolonged physical and cognitive inactivity, the so-called cocoon therapy. New data have shown that rest exceeding 3 days is not likely to be helpful or can even be harmful and that gradual return to preinjury activities should begin as soon as tolerated.[35] Studies have even shown that early and controlled exercise that does not exacerbate symptoms may have some potential in preventing postconcussive symptoms as well as reducing the risk of developing a mood or anxiety disorder.[36]

Conversely, premature return to activity can exacerbate concussion symptoms or prolong recovery.[37] The risks can be grave and include increased probability of sustaining another concussion at a lower impact level, prolonged recovery time, and/or precipitation of mood and anxiety disorders. DeMatteo and colleagues recommend the following in order to mitigate premature RTP, specifically in youth populations:

- No contact sport for 3 months in the event of positive neuroimaging.
- No contact sport for 6 months if there have been 2 concussions within 3 months.
- Removal from contact sports for 1 year if there have been 3 concussions within 1 year.[34]

These recommendations were based on the principal that existing protocols are not specific to youth athletes and that more conservative management may be indicated in this demographic.

In addition to the physical and mental long-term risks, athletes who have experienced concussion may also experience a level of stigmatization. Studies have demonstrated that individuals may experience pressure to suppress or minimize concussion-related symptoms,[38] and this can be intentional (an athlete trying to return to activity prematurely) or unintentional (not understanding the implications of this action). Sources of pressure include the athlete themselves, coaches, teammates, parents, media, and fans.[39]

The Impact of Removal from Sport

There are considerable implications regarding removal from sport for any reason. For instance, Mainwaring and colleagues found that National Collegiate Athletic Association football players with anterior cruciate ligament injury endorsed higher levels of depression and for longer periods of time than those who had experienced

Table 1
Graduated return-to-sport strategy

Stage	Aim	Activity	Goal of Each Step
1	Symptom-limited activity	Daily activities that do not provoke symptoms	Gradual reintroduction of work/school activities
2	Light aerobic exercise	Walking or stationary cycling at slow to medium pace. No resistance training	Increase heart rate
3	Sport-specific exercise	Running or skating drills. No head-impact activities	Add movement
4	Noncontact training drills	Harder training drills, for example, passing drills. May start progressive resistance training	Exercise, coordination, and increased thinking
5	Full-contact practice	Following medical clearance, participate in normal training activities	Restore confidence and assess functional skills by coaching staff
6	Return to sport	Normal game play	

NOTE: An initial period of 24–48 h of both relative physical rest and cognitive rest is recommended before beginning the RTS progression. There should be at least 24 h (or longer) for each step of the progression. If any symptoms worsen during exercise, the athlete should go back to the previous step. Resistance training should be added only in the later stages (stage 3 or 4 at the earliest). If symptoms are persistent (eg, more than 10–14 d in adults or more than 1 mo in children), the athlete should be referred to a health care professional who is an expert in the management of concussion.

Stage	Aim	Activity	Goal of Each Step
1	Daily activities at home that do not give the child symptoms	Typical activities of the child during the day as long as they do not increase symptoms (eg, reading, texting, screen time). Start with 5–15 min at a time and gradually build up	Gradual return to typical activities
2	School activities	Homework, reading, or other cognitive activities outside of the classroom	Increase tolerance to cognitive work
3	Return to school part-time	Gradual introduction of schoolwork. May need to start with a partial school day or with increased breaks during the day	Increase academic activities
4	Return to school full time	Gradually progress school activities until a full day can be tolerated	Return to full academic activities and catch up on missed work

Abbreviation: RTS, return to sport.
From McCrory P, Meeuwisse W, Dvorak J, et al Consensus statement on concussion in sport—the 5th international conference on concussion in sport held in Berlin, October 2016 British Journal of Sports Medicine 2017;51:838-847, with permission.

Table 2 Contraindication to return to sport	
Relative Contraindications	**Absolute Contraindication**
• History of postconcussive symptoms that are present at the time of evaluation or >90 d • Cognitive impairment • Diminished academic performance or social engagement • Decreased concussion threshold	• Evidence of structural brain injury after TBI • Structural abnormalities associated with increased risk of hemorrhage

Data from Davis-Hayes C, Baker DR, Bottiglieri TS, et al. Medical retirement from sport after concussions: A practical guide for a difficult discussion. *Neurology Clinical practice.* 2018;8(1):40-47.

concussion.[40] It is known that physical activity can have both biological and psychological benefits including increased self-confidence, improved mood, decreased symptoms of depression and anxiety, and improvements to one's overall sense of well-being.[41,42] Removal from sport can be expected to lead to a range of responses mediated by biological, psychological, and social factors (**Table 3**).

At a biological level, removal from sport has the potential to lead to neurochemical and other physical changes that may affect mood. Aerobic exercise has been demonstrated to increase production of endogenous opiates and improve one's sense of well-being.[43] The abrupt cessation of routine physical activity leading to a decrease in the positive neurochemical benefits of sport has the potential to perpetuate or even precipitate a depressive episode. Removal from sport due to concussion has the added implications of neurochemical imbalance and other neuroinflammatory processes.

At a psychological level, injuries or experiences that lead to removal from sport may be extremely threatening to an athlete. Athletes frequently spend considerable time and effort maintaining peak physicality, but even a minor injury may challenge this. As a result, they may question their sense of physical integrity and identity as an athlete, leading to a degree of distress and potentially even trauma.[44] A sense of responsibility to one's family and athletic community can also influence the development of a trauma response.[45] It has been demonstrated that psychosocial factors have the potential to significantly affect recovery from any injury.[46] In particular, fear of reinjury

Table 3 Potential impacts of sport-related concussion		
Biological	**Psychological**	**Social**
• Neurochemical Cascade of concussion • Neuroinflammation • Somatic symptoms (headache, nausea, dizziness, etc.) • Deconditioning from inactivity • Disruption of neuroendocrine benefits of sport due to inactivity	• Cognitive dysfunction • Worry about future concussion/reinjury • Disruption to a sense of physicality, threat to bodily integrity • Stress response or posttraumatic stress disorder	• Removal from the team setting • Guilt about not contributing to the team due to injury • Worry about academics • Worry about career or scholarship • Shame experienced due to having an "invisible injury"

is one of the most common emotional factors experienced by an athlete and may interfere with recovery and engagement in rehabilitation.[47]

The psychosocial benefits of participating in sport are manifold and may be even more pronounced with participation in team sports that requires a higher level of collaboration with peers. With socialization in sport, one may see an improved self-esteem and increased feelings of interconnectedness.[48,49] Removal of these beneficial aspects of socialization can be considerable and may leave an athlete feeling isolated with experiences such as shame, guilt, or depression. To mitigate this, an athlete should be allowed to engage in nonexertional team-based activities, meetings, and gatherings as tolerated.[50]

EVALUATING SPORT-RELATED CONCUSSION–RELATED RETIREMENT
Retirement

There is currently no medical consensus or guideline regarding when SRC should lead to retirement from a sport or transition to a new sport. This conversation can be extremely delicate and may have considerable implications for those competing at an elite level. Many providers have adhered to the "3-strike rule" where an individual who has experienced 3 concussions should be considered ineligible to return to sport[51]; this can be attributed to Thorndike who in 1952 noted that after "…three concussions, which involved loss of consciousness for any period of time, the athlete should be removed from contact sports for the remainder of the season."[52] However, this was the investigator's opinion based on research examining individuals with a range of mild to severe TBI. Ultimately, we do not have any empirical basis for adherence to the "3-strike rule" or any other rigid guidelines regarding mandated retirement. As such, it is recommended that exploration of retirement due to SRC takes place on an individualized basis.

A discussion about retirement can be considered if there is evidence of concerning or severe neurologic disturbance, significantly decreased concussion threshold, or persistent symptoms that have negatively affected an athlete's life.[33] It is prudent that the physician begins with an assessment of current injury status, performs an evaluation of future risk of injury, and considers clinical decision modifiers in addition to what the athlete views as personal decision modifiers.[39] Conducting a risk-benefit analysis is a modifiable and personalized approach that attempts to minimize any conscious or personal biases. By following a structured conversation, there is less room for personal subjectivity to interfere with such a life-changing decision, which can also lead to a discussion about transitioning to a lower risk sport depending on persistent symptoms and risk factors.

Retirement for athletes can be a difficult life transition and is the most important risk factor for suicide in professional athletes.[53] Many competitive athletes who are highly invested in their sport feel defined by their participation and status level. Approaching this topic with an athlete is therefore critical, yet sensitive, as it threatens the perceived and experienced athletic identity. Regardless of whether the athlete retires in a "normative" or "nonnormative" way, they will typically experience a wide range of psychological, interpersonal, and financial changes.[54]

A WAY FORWARD

Although efforts to improve the safety of sport through changes in equipment and modifications to existing rules and regulations have been meaningful, the occurrence of SRC nonetheless persists. Regardless of the gaps in our understanding of SRC, every effort should be made to ensure that participation in youth sport is a safe and positive experience for everyone involved.

Efforts to target this are multifaceted and require collaboration across disciplines. Coaches, trainers, and parents play an important role in fostering the psychosocial benefits associated with a safe sporting experience, as well as a meaningful recovery in the event of SRC. For providers, it is critical to provide psychoeducation using empirical evidence. It can be beneficial to share the strengths and weaknesses regarding the current understanding of this type of injury, given the prevalence of misconceptions regarding SRC. The potential benefits of sport participation should be emphasized and balanced against the risks. Participation in any activity involving a degree of physicality has the potential for injury, though it should be stressed that a sedentary lifestyle has the potential to be equally, if not more damaging.[55]

Although efforts have been made to create a "one-size-fits-all" template for management of SRC, concussion is a heterogenous injury with numerous factors that have the potential to affect recovery. Any treatment should be tailored to the individual with a focus on both preexisting conditions and persistent symptoms, as well as the psychosocial factors that can either perpetuate or promote a recovery.

SUMMARY

Participation in sport at the youth level has tremendous benefit on multiple levels and is invaluable in creating a healthy and active population. Although our understanding of SRC continues to evolve, efforts should be made to ensure a safe experience that enhances youth sport engagement. SRC can affect an individual in a range of biological and psychosocial ways. Careful consideration of these factors is imperative in order to ensure a meaningful recovery and return to sport.

CLINICS CARE POINTS

- Concussion can impact an athlete in ways that are unique compared to non-athletes.
- Careful consideration of biological, psychological, and social factors is crucial when helping an athlete navigate recovery from SRC.
- Appropriate psychoeducation for players, family, coaches, and teammates, is important to avoid certain pitfalls that may complicate recovery from SRC.
- Media portrayal of SRC, including reports on scientific literature, can be complicated and may be a source of confusion for individuals who experience SRC.
- Psychopharmacological interventions can be considered if SRC-related symptoms do not improve within a reasonable course of time, and with careful consideration of the risks and benefits specific to each individual athlete.

DISCLOSURE

The authors have nothing to disclose.

REFERENCES

1. Martland HS. Punch drunk. J Am Med Assoc 1927;91:1103–7.
2. McCrory P, Meeuwisse W, Dvorak J, et al. Consensus statement on concussion in sport-the 5th international conference on concussion in sport held in Berlin, October 2016. Br J Sports Med 2017;51(11):838–47.

3. Giza CC, Hovda DA. The neurometabolic cascade of concussion. J Athl Train 2001;36(3):228–35.

4. Giza CC, Hovda DA. The new neurometabolic cascade of concussion. Neurosurgery 2014;75(Suppl 4):S24–33.

5. Langlois JA, Rutland-Brown W, Wald MM. The epidemiology and impact of traumatic brain injury: a brief overview. J Head Trauma Rehabil 2006;21(5):375–8.

6. Coronado V, McGuire L, Faul M, et al. Traumatic brain injury epidemiology and public health issues. In: Brain injury medicine: principles and practice. New York, NY: Demos Medical Publishing; 2012. p. 84–100.

7. Gilchrist J, Thomas K, Xu L, et al. Centers for disease control and prevention: Nonfatal traumatic brain injuries related traumatic brain injuries among children and adolescents treated in emergency departments in the United States, 2001-2009. MMWR Morb Mortal Wkly Rep 2011;60(39):1337–42.

8. Lincoln AE, Caswell SV, Almquist JL, et al. Trends in concussion incidence in high school sports: a prospective 11-year study. Am J Sports Med 2011;39(5):958–63.

9. Pfister T, Pfister K, Hagel B, et al. The incidence of concussion in youth sports: a systematic review and meta-analysis. Br J Sports Med 2016;50(5):292–7.

10. Associations NFoSHS. Participation in high school sports registers first decline in 30 years. 2019. Available at: https://www.nfhs.org/articles/participation-in-high-school-sports-registers-first-decline-in-30-years/. Accessed August 24, 2020.

11. Media S. SFIA: sports industry facing too many casual participants. 2019. Available at: https://sgbonline.com/sfia-industry-has-too-many-casual-partiicpants/. Accessed August 24, 2020.

12. Farrey T. ESPN poll: most parents have concerns about state of youth sports. 2014. Available at: https://www.espn.com/espnw/w-in-action/story/_/id/11675649/parents-concern-grows-kids-participation-sports. Accessed August 21, 2020.

13. UPMC. How knowledgeable are americans about concussions? Assessing and recalibrating the public's knowledge. 2015. Available at: https://rethinkconcussions.upmc.com/wp-content/uploads/2015/09/harris-poll-report.pdf. Accessed August 31, 2020.

14. Ku C, McKinlay A, Grace RC, et al. An international exploration of the effect of media portrayals of postconcussion management on concussion identification in the general public. J Head Trauma Rehabil 2020;35(3):218–25.

15. Andrikopoulos J. Age of first exposure to football and later-life cognitive impairment in former NFL players. Neurology 2015;85(11):1007.

16. Stamm JM, Bourlas AP, Baugh CM, et al. Age of first exposure to football and later-life cognitive impairment in former NFL players. Neurology 2015;84(11):1114–20.

17. Alosco ML, Kasimis AB, Stamm JM, et al. Age of first exposure to American football and long-term neuropsychiatric and cognitive outcomes. Transl Psychiatry 2017;7(9):e1236.

18. Solomon GS, Kuhn AW, Zuckerman SL, et al. Participation in pre-high school football and neurological, neuroradiological, and neuropsychological findings in later life: a study of 45 retired national football league players. Am J Sports Med 2016;44(5):1106–15.

19. Janssen PH, Mandrekar J, Mielke MM, et al. High school football and late-life risk of neurodegenerative syndromes, 1956-1970. Mayo Clin Proc 2017;92(1):66–71.

20. Brett BL, Huber DL, Wild A, et al. Age of first exposure to american football and behavioral, cognitive, psychological, and physical outcomes in high school and collegiate football players. Sports Health 2019;11(4):332–42.

21. Caccese JB, Iverson GL, Cameron KL, et al. Estimated age of first exposure to contact sports is not associated with greater symptoms or worse cognitive functioning in male U.S. service academy athletes. J Neurotrauma 2020;37(2):334–9.
22. Savica R, Parisi JE, Wold LE, et al. High school football and risk of neurodegeneration: a community-based study. Mayo Clin Proc 2012;87(4):335–40.
23. Zuckerman SL, Brett BL, Jeckell AS, et al. Prognostic factors in pediatric sport-related concussion. Curr Neurol Neurosci Rep 2018;18(12):104.
24. Omalu BI, DeKosky ST, Minster RL, et al. Chronic traumatic encephalopathy in a National Football League player. Neurosurgery 2005;57(1):128–34, discussion 128–134.
25. Mez J, Daneshvar DH, Kiernan PT, et al. Clinicopathological evaluation of chronic traumatic encephalopathy in players of American football. JAMA 2017;318(4): 360–70.
26. Ward J, Williams J, Manchester S. 110 N.F.L. Brains. New York Times 2017.
27. Gardner A, Iverson GL, McCrory P. Chronic traumatic encephalopathy in sport: a systematic review. Br J Sports Med 2014;48(2):84–90.
28. Solomon GS, Zuckerman SL. Chronic traumatic encephalopathy in professional sports: retrospective and prospective views. Brain Inj 2015;29(2):164–70.
29. Kuhn AW, Yengo-Kahn AM, Kerr ZY, et al. Sports concussion research, chronic traumatic encephalopathy and the media: repairing the disconnect. Br J Sports Med 2017;51(24):1732–3.
30. Stewart W, Allinson K, Al-Sarraj S, et al. Primum non nocere: a call for balance when reporting on CTE. Lancet Neurol 2019;18(3):231–3.
31. Halstead ME, Walter KD, Moffatt K. Sport-related concussion in children and adolescents. Pediatrics 2018;142(6):e20183074.
32. Meehan WP 3rd. Medical therapies for concussion. Clin Sports Med 2011;30(1): 115–24, ix.
33. Davis-Hayes C, Baker DR, Bottiglieri TS, et al. Medical retirement from sport after concussions: a practical guide for a difficult discussion. Neurol Clin Pract 2018; 8(1):40–7.
34. DeMatteo C, Stazyk K, Singh SK, et al. Development of a conservative protocol to return children and youth to activity following concussive injury. Clin Pediatr 2014; 54(2):152–63.
35. Silverberg ND, Iverson GL. Is rest after concussion "the best medicine?": recommendations for activity resumption following concussion in athletes, civilians, and military service members. J Head Trauma Rehabil 2013;28(4):250–9.
36. Leddy JJ, Wilber CG, Willer BS. Active recovery from concussion. Curr Opin Neurol 2018;31(6):681–6.
37. Carson JD, Lawrence DW, Kraft SA, et al. Premature return to play and return to learn after a sport-related concussion: physician's chart review. Can Fam Physician 2014;60(6):e310, e312-315.
38. Lininger M, Wayment HA, Huffman AH, et al. An exploratory study on concussion-reporting behaviors from collegiate student athletes' perspectives. Athletic Train Sports Health Care 2017;9:71–80.
39. Kroshus E, Garnett B, Hawrilenko M, et al. Concussion under-reporting and pressure from coaches, teammates, fans, and parents. Soc Sci Med 2015;134:66–75.
40. Mainwaring LM, Hutchison M, Bisschop SM, et al. Emotional response to sport concussion compared to ACL injury. Brain Inj 2010;24(4):589–97.
41. Eime RM, Young JA, Harvey JT, et al. A systematic review of the psychological and social benefits of participation in sport for children and adolescents:

informing development of a conceptual model of health through sport. Int J Behav Nutr Phys Act 2013;10:98.

42. Guddal MH, Stensland S, Småstuen MC, et al. Physical activity and sport participation among adolescents: associations with mental health in different age groups. Results from the Young-HUNT study: a cross-sectional survey. BMJ Open 2019;9(9):e028555.

43. Kraemer WJ, Dziados JE, Marchitelli LJ, et al. Effects of different heavy-resistance exercise protocols on plasma beta-endorphin concentrations. J Appl Physiol (1985) 1993;74(1):450–9.

44. Brassil HE, Salvatore AP. The frequency of post-traumatic stress disorder symptoms in athletes with and without sports related concussion. Clin Transl Med 2018;7(1):25.

45. Wenzel T, Zhu LJ. Posttraumatic stress in athletes. United Kingdom: Wiley; 2013.

46. Forsdyke D, Smith A, Jones M, et al. Psychosocial factors associated with outcomes of sports injury rehabilitation in competitive athletes: a mixed studies systematic review. Br J Sports Med 2016;50(9):537–44.

47. Ardern CL, Taylor NF, Feller JA, et al. A systematic review of the psychological factors associated with returning to sport following injury. Br J Sports Med 2013;47(17):1120–6.

48. Boone EM, Leadbeater BJ. Game on: Diminishing risks for depressive symptoms in early adolescence through positive involvement in team sports. J Res Adolescence 2006;16(1):79–90.

49. Pedersen S, Seidman E. Team sports achievement and self-esteem development among urban adolescent girls. Psychol Women Quart 2004;28(4):412–22.

50. Schneider KJ, Iverson GL, Emery CA, et al. The effects of rest and treatment following sport-related concussion: a systematic review of the literature. Br J Sports Med 2013;47(5):304–7.

51. McCrory P. When to retire after concussion? Br J Sports Med 2001;35(6):380–2.

52. Thorndike A. Serious recurrent injuries of athletes; contraindications to further competitive participation. N Engl J Med 1952;247(15):554–6.

53. Brown GT, Hainline B, Kroshus E, et al. Mind, body and sport: understanding and supporting student-athlete mental wellness. Indianapolis, IN: National Collegiate Athletic Association; 2014.

54. Knights S, Sherry E, Ruddock-Hudson M. Investigating elite end-of-athletic-career transition: a systematic review. J Appl Sport Psychol 2016;28(3):291–308.

55. Hoare E, Milton K, Foster C, et al. The associations between sedentary behaviour and mental health among adolescents: a systematic review. Int J Behav Nutr Phys Act 2016;13(1):108.

Selection/Interview Criteria for Drafting Players

David Putrino, PT, PhD[a],*, Paul H. Groenewal, PsyD[b], Rosemarie Perry, PhD[c,d]

KEYWORDS

- Athlete performance • Talent identification • Talent selection • Draft selection

KEY POINTS

- There is currently no gold-standard metric, or aggregate of metrics, for predicting future performance of an athlete in a draft setting.
- Understanding the environmental, physical, and psychological context surrounding draft performance for each athlete is crucial to successful talent identification and selection.
- Every effort should be made to create objective data collection frameworks for drafting protocols so that decisions are data-driven and less prone to confounds and implicit bias.
- High performance is as influenced by environmental conditions as it is by more traditionally measured athlete-level performance indicators, such as cognitive and perceptual skill sets.
- During player selection assessments, sports organizations should evaluate for "performance fit": the fit between a player's performance styles and the performance demands of the sporting environment.

INTRODUCTION: PHYSICAL COMPETENCY AND PERFORMANCE

The use of the term "draft" to define the procedure of selecting a group of high performers highlights the influence that military selection protocols has historically had on athlete selection procedures. Military protocols continue to deeply influence drafting in sports performance, and given this influence, a physical draft remains one of the most important elements for decision making in many professional sports teams. As such, all professional sports teams conduct a team-specific physical draft and usually participate in a predraft "Combine" involving coaches, scouts, and other interested parties, to identify favorable sports-specific skills and attributes in prospective players. These assessments typically include measurement of muscle strength, endurance, physical features (such as height, body fat percentage, and arm span), and sport-specific hard skills. Physical drafting protocols vary widely across different

[a] Department of Rehabilitation and Human Performance, Icahn School of Medicine at Mount Sinai, 1 Gustave L. Levy Pl, Box 1240, New York, NY 10029, USA; [b] Inspire Wellness, Glen Rock, NJ, USA; [c] Social Creatures, Brooklyn, NY, USA; [d] Department of Applied Psychology, New York University, New York, NY, USA
* Corresponding author.
E-mail address: david.putrino@mountsinai.org

Psychiatr Clin N Am 44 (2021) 481–492
https://doi.org/10.1016/j.psc.2021.04.012
0193-953X/21/© 2021 Elsevier Inc. All rights reserved.
psych.theclinics.com

sports because the physical attributes that are favorable for optimal performance in each sport also vary widely. Notably, physical screening procedures hold high predictive value in a military selection environment whereby selection is occurring from a normative pool of applicants, and performance prediction is graded as a binary, pass/fail construct.[1,2] However, in a professional sports environment, where applicants are selected from a smaller pool of existing high performers with similar sets of physical attributes, the predictive validity of physical screening procedures on performance remains questionable.[3] Thus, although physical attributes and competencies are helpful "pass/fail" screening tools to use on prospective players, sports organizations should recognize that these attributes and competencies do not reliably translate to player performance.

SCOUTING HIGH PERFORMERS

In professional sports, it is acknowledged that objective metrics of performance can only partially inform the talent selection process.[4] Even sports such as American Football, which has shown correlations between objective performances at the NFL Combine and draft pick status, have not demonstrated a similar relationship between draft pick status and career performance.[5,6] Thus, an important part of talent selection is knowledge regarding a prospective athlete's in-context performance of their sport, data that are beyond the restrictive nature of artificially created objective testing. Observation and reporting of these in-context performances are the domain of talent scouts, who traditionally serve as an important source of information for the talent selection process. Despite the important role that scouts play in the talent identification and recruitment process, there is very little described in the literature about their specific process in identifying talent. Certainly, much of the scouting process is performed subjectively; individuals with deep knowledge and experience with the sport travel from location to location and observe players of interest as they engage in local games and competitions. Trusted scouts will typically have a vast network of connections that provide them with "intelligence" on up-and-coming players who may have potential for professional competition. In addition to information about performance on the field, scouts also work to gather information about off-field metrics, such as general coachability, family life, and other socially pertinent factors that may influence a player's ability to perform in a new environment. A crucial expectation of scouts is to have a detailed understanding of the difference between high performance in a lower-tier competition and high performance in a professional sports setting. For instance, many of the factors that make a collegiate athlete a great performer may not hold when they are given an opportunity to perform on a national level. It is an expectation that a scout can identify and differentiate players that can successfully make this transition, and those who may struggle.

Talent scouts have a difficult task to complete. Although there is increasing pressure to make the scouting process more objective across many professional sports, the fact remains that much of the important information being gathered and relayed by scouts is largely subjective. Reliance on subjective data leads to many inherent biases in the scouting process, and all members of a performance team should be mindful that these biases exist because they can lead to talent wastage and reduced efficacy of talent selection.[7] The following 3 major forms of bias have been reported in the field of talent selection:

1. *Racial stacking bias:* Racial stacking, a propensity for scouts to favor athletes of certain races in certain positions (such as white quarterbacks in American football

or black outfielders in baseball), has existed in professional sports for many years.[8] Although inroads have been made to begin to address this issue in many sports, it is still a source of significant unconscious bias in subjective assessment of performance and is a major source of talent wastage.

2. *Sunk-cost bias:* Scouting for talent is a difficult and time-consuming process, and many scouts will often have to follow a player of interest to many games, involving a good amount of commitment and travel. This can lead to another form of bias known as the "sunk-cost bias": if a talent scout has been "chasing" a prospective athlete for longer than usual or has gained information that was particularly difficult to acquire, it may lead to a tendency to oversell the athlete in order to get a "return on the investment" of time and energy.[7]

3. *Tacit knowledge bias:* Talent scouts are typically former athletes or coaches, and their lived experiences are incredibly valuable for cultivating a skilled "eye" for talent identification. However, their tacit knowledge, the knowledge they acquired through such former experience, can influence their judgment of player performance, creating a level of bias that should be taken into consideration.[9] For instance, an American football talent scout that used to play as a quarterback may judge other quarterbacks more harshly, and other positions less harshly. If the selection team is unaware of this bias, it can lead to inaccuracies in the way that they rank athlete reports coming in from different scouts.

ORIGINS OF PSYCHOLOGICAL AND COGNITIVE DRAFTING PROCEDURES

Professional sports organizations increasingly understand that sustained individual and team performance is driven by more than an athlete's physical competency; psychological factors and cognitive competencies are also necessary to maintain elite athletic performance. Thus, many teams have worked to become more sophisticated in their approaches toward talent selection, developing criteria that evaluate an athlete beyond their simple physical competencies. In developing these criteria, many professional sports organizations find themselves once again turning to military procedure, especially as it pertains to special forces training, to identify some psychological features of high performers that may translate to high performance in athletes. For instance, research on elite warfighters has identified resilience, self-efficacy, grit, hardiness, and internal locus of control as favorable attributes that are predictive of high-performing special forces operators, highlighting the potential value in investigating these psychological domains during athlete drafting and screening procedures.[10,11] Mindset has also been explored as an important predictor of performance in elite military, with results painting a nuanced picture of the influence of mindset on elite performance. For instance, in a study of 174 Navy SEAL candidates, it was shown that adopting a positive mindset around stress ("stress is enhancing") resulted in higher performance, but a positive mindset around failure ("failure is enhancing") was detrimental to performance.[12] Findings such as these highlight the complexity and nuance that sports organizations must consider around the psychology of high performance when assessing prospective players. Ultimately, the research around the psychology of high performance in the elite warfighter literature can serve as a good starting point for sports performance organizations that are interested in developing their own frameworks for psychological selection criteria. However, professional sports organizations should be cautioned about attempting to closely emulate the military literature and experience when creating their psychological drafting protocols: warfighting is not the same as professional sports performance, and thus, talent selection protocols should similarly differ.

PSYCHOLOGICAL DRAFTING: BEST PRACTICES IN SPORTS PERFORMANCE

There are numerous considerations for establishing a psychological drafting procedure that is complementary and additive to the overall talent selection process, while controlling for the risk of creating an inaccurate or unfair view of the athlete or creating a negative perception of the selection process. If this is not well achieved, it can significantly impact the extent to which selected athletes feel comfortable or safe using the Sport Psychology/Psychiatry services offered by the team.

KNOW WHAT IS BEING MEASURED FOR PLAYER ASSESSMENTS

The first step of the psychological drafting process is completing a job analysis to guide the assessment protocol and development of player selection criteria. Job analyses, which identify the important components and elements of a position to be filled, are frequently conducted in nonsporting industries to maximize the effectiveness of employee selection processes. In fact, in accordance with human resource management best practices, conducting a job analysis is the first step toward identifying the specific constructs (eg, cognitive ability, interpersonal skills) that should be assessed in the selection process.[13] It may not be possible to complete a structured job analysis within every sports organization; however, developing a clear picture of the organization's perceived needs and, more specifically, the "job" or position that they are attempting to fill greatly aids the selection process. It clarifies which measures can be used to select for players and, more specifically, which data points are most relevant for selection. Furthermore, using human resource management practices to develop and communicate selection criteria to prospective players is vital to ensuring a fair and equitable selection process.[14]

A thorough selection process that includes objective and subjective data gathered in a structured way is the most effective.[14,15] It reduces bias and provides an objective way to compare athletes. Barrick and colleagues[16] found that interviews (especially if unstructured) were prone to self-presentation tactics, and that interview-collected data did not necessarily translate to job performance. Objective assessment can help those involved in the selection process control for bias and impression management. It is essential to educate the stakeholders on both the value of the objective data and the limitations; this is especially true in selecting for sport. Although there are no current measures that show clear evidence of predicting performance levels, predicting high performers is often the referral question.

ESTABLISH CLEAR EXPECTATIONS FOR HOW ASSESSMENT INFORMATION WILL BE COMMUNICATED

When it comes to conducting player assessments, psychologists/psychiatrists should be sure to communicate up front when meeting with each athlete that their "client" is the sports organization, which is typically the case for the selection process. Psychologists/psychiatrists should also indicate the organization's desire for the assessment and the intent to interpret the data that assist in the selection process. This explanation should also include the boundaries involved, such as not providing the raw data to the organization and not providing information outside of what is necessary for the selection process. Human resource management literature discusses the lack of training managers receive in psychometric properties, highlighting the need for assessment measures to be interpreted with care by a trained professional. Managers are unlikely to be fully aware of the constructs being assessed, including the potential limitations. Thus, without expert guidance, they are likely to draw inaccurate and possibly unfair conclusions when using assessment measures for selection.[17] For personality measures, as an example, it is best practice to provide a partial profile focused only on the personality characteristics relevant to the position and culture fit with the broader organization. The lack of training in psychometrics is true for most sports organizations as well, the general managers and staff do not have training in psychometrics; therefore, the data must be obtained and provided in a way that benefits their selection process while at the same time protecting from misinterpretation or the misuse of the data.

When communicating findings with the stakeholders of the organization, psychologists/psychiatrists should be cognizant of the language used, avoiding clinical language that may be misused or increase stigma, such as "crazy" or "sociopath." The framing of information can have negative implications for years to come in terms of how the organization, and those who are close to the organization, views the player. That perception could have career-altering implications. The context of behaviors witnessed is also a vital consideration in avoiding judgment/bias. Is the player using sarcasm to engage staff, or is it a signal that he/she is disrespectful and passive-aggressive? Psychologists/psychiatrists should consider all possibilities and allow objective data to guide their assessments. If witnessing behaviors that would influence the overall assessment, it can be helpful to follow up. For instance, if a player rolls his eyes when a physical therapist asks him/her to complete a movement, it may be an immature attempt to connect rather than a blatant attempt to show his/her displeasure with the request. Asking the athlete about the interaction and their intent can help determine the significance of behavior and provides useful data that could shed light on the player's interpersonal tendencies, level of maturity, self-awareness, and social skills.

DETERMINE HOW THE ASSESSMENT INFORMATION WILL BE USED INTERNALLY

There must also be considerations for how the assessment information will benefit the athlete that is selected. Knowing what was needed to gain selection will provide a clearer understanding of the organization's values and what the organization expects from athletes. If, for instance, an athlete knew they were selected for their high character and their ability to problem solve quickly, they are more likely to invest in opportunities that display their strength of character and to engage in opportunities that prepare them to problem solve during competitions. Indeed, theoretic work and empirical work have highlighted the positive impact of assessment on therapeutic outcomes.[18,19] In sports organizations, this means that the assessment data obtained during selection could easily be related to the growth organizations want to see in their athletes. Once an athlete is selected, the organization is likely invested in that athlete, furthering their personal and professional development, rather than selecting them with no expectation for growth or change. Therefore, the assessment information can identify strengths, weaknesses, and strategies for growth. The athlete can use these strengths, weaknesses, and strategies to increase self-awareness, including clear recommendations for personal and professional growth.

DETERMINING PSYCHOLOGICAL ASSESSMENTS FOR PLAYER SELECTION

In conducting player talent identification and selection, sport organizations routinely incorporate psychological assessments to aid identification and selection of high performing athletes. However, determining how psychological assessments are used for player selection should be driven by an organization's unique culture and criteria for high performance and be informed by a clear understanding of the strengths and limitations that psychological assessments provide.

Defining High Performance

First and foremost, the successful use of psychological assessments hinges on the recruiting organization's ability to first define their "constructs of interest" clearly, that is, the psychological indicators that they will evaluate as markers of "high performance" for each prospective player. However, there is not yet an exact science that can be applied to select for high performers. Across sports, both researchers and practitioners acknowledge that psychological drivers of athletic performance are multidimensional and can involve cognitive and perceptual capabilities, mental skills and strategies, as well as interpersonal skills.[20–23] However, it is important that organizations ultimately choose to assess constructs that most closely align with their predetermined criteria for high performance and the unique demands of the sporting context in which players will be performing.

This need to contextualize construct selection is driven by commonly documented validity issues with psychological testing batteries in player selection scenarios. Indeed, although psychological testing batteries afford several strengths, their strengths must be weighed against their limitations when used in applied athletic settings. Psychological testing batteries provide the strength of assessing constructs of interest in a highly structured format, enabling quantitative data collection that is far less influenced by the biases and confounding influences that commonly plague unstructured scout and staff evaluations.[4,24–26] However, no existing psychometrics or other objective psychological assessments have been well validated as reliable predictors of subsequent athlete performance levels.[27] The low predictive validity of common psychological testing batteries is concomitant with, and likely driven by, their issues with ecological validity. Psychological assessments and testing batteries do not correlate strongly with actual athlete performance in context, nor do they typically accurately represent sport demands.[28,29]

The identification of constructs and development of assessment tools that can reliably delineate elite performers remain an active and ongoing area of research in sports psychology. However, these efforts will likely prove unsuccessful unless disagreements around the definition and theoretic underpinnings of athletic talent and performance are first resolved. Although athletic talent is traditionally defined as an exceptional natural ability to perform a sports-related task or activity, it is increasingly recognized that talent cannot be disentangled from context.[21,28,30] Indeed, the ability to optimally perform is directly influenced by dynamic situational factors, and this includes the environment and social context in which one is performing, as well as broader ecological factors, such as socioeconomic, threat, and deprivation factors, that can deeply influence the development and opportunities for expression of "talent" (eg, Refs.[31,32]). For instance, player abilities that are thought to play a significant role in athletic success, such as cognitive and motor skills, develop *through* dynamic interactions with the environment (eg, Refs.[33–36]). Furthermore, the extent to which the same skills contribute to successful performance is increasingly recognized to vary across situational factors, such as across different sporting domains, levels of competitions, playing positions, and ages of athletes.[37] Thus, the theoretic mechanism underlying athletic talent, and ultimately high performance, can be characterized by the development and interrelation of skills that are contextually embedded.[21,29,30]

Collectively, this advancement in empirical and theoretic research challenges the assumption that athletic talent is a fixed capacity that is stable across time, rather supporting that talent is continuously developed and gated through the dynamic influence of a network of contextual factors. This implies that the environment and situational factors, including demands of the performance environment, as well as the role of coaches, staff, and even family members, can override the natural ability of the performer, for better or worse.[38–40] Taken together, this further supports the need to contextualize the construct selection and assessment process in drafts. Unless sport organizations fully recognize their inherent contextual influence on player performance, they will not be optimizing for high performance. As such, organizations should optimize their psychological assessments for high performance by making every attempt to assess player performance within the environments in which they will be performing, keeping player-environment interactions intact during assessment procedures. The authors refer to the concerted measurement of athlete-level and context-level factors as the assessment of "performance fit," whereby organizations seek to assess the "fit" between a player's performance styles and performance demands of the operating environment (**Fig. 1**).

Assessing Performance Fit

The successful identification of psychological constructs for the assessment of performance fit requires highly interactive and sustained collaboration between a sports organization's management team, staff, psychologists/psychiatrists, and data scientists. Indicators of performance fit should not follow a "one-size-fits-all" approach, but rather be selected on a basis that is specific to the organization's sport, culture, team, and staff dynamics, all through the lens of the specific position to be filled. Where possible, this includes, structured, data-driven assessment of an athlete's psychological performance characteristics across contexts and situational factors deemed most relevant to gameplay and the sports organization's culture and environmental demands. Such assessment of performance fit can manifest in several ways. Organizations can work directly with scouts to insert a data-driven approach to their standard evaluations of player performance. Draft procedures can prioritize in-house psychological assessments that involve interactions with existing staff and/or

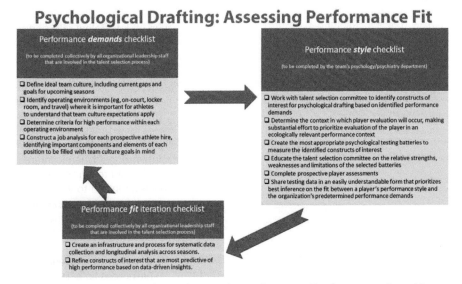

Fig. 1. An iterative checklist for evaluating the performance fit of a prospective athlete.

teammates. Psychological testing batteries that are well validated to measure specific characteristics or skills can be used to assess player attitudes, beliefs, and mental strategies that are consistent with the organization's predetermined mission, culture, and high-performance values. The authors encourage organizations to incorporate academically rigorous assessment and evaluation methodology used in social and developmental psychology (eg, dyadic and social network analyses), fields that focus on the assessment and development of human behavior and performance within broader social and environmental contexts. However, regardless of the methodology that an organization chooses to use, the central goal should remain to conduct psychological assessments in the most structured and data-driven manner possible, reducing confounds and biases in the assessment and eventual decision making around player recruitment.

Notably, the successful assessment of performance fit is predicated on the sports organization first defining and protecting their own organizational values and norms, team culture, and staff/player roles and responsibilities. As such, significant efforts should be placed on the deliberate crafting and maintenance of organizational culture, rules, norms, and protocols before player assessments are designed and initiated. For instance, will the organization treat athletic talent as a fixed trait, or recognize talent as the expression of dynamic skill sets that are continually influenced and developed through context? What level of staff and team bonding will be expected of athletes, and how are they expected to conduct themselves within these social scenarios? What types of pressure should players anticipate in their performance environments and unique playing position, at what frequency, intensity, and duration? How will organizational staff lead and manage each player? What is the manner and context in which staff beliefs and attitudes about the players will be conveyed? What types of familial sacrifices, if any, will the organization expect players to make to engage in their sport across the season? Will the organization be drafting players into an environment of holistic player care, providing structured and reliable physical, emotional, nutritional, and financial support? Predetermining situational factors such as these will ultimately guide what psychological testing batteries will be most appropriate for the performance fit assessment of prospective players and staff.

Finally, the successful design of performance fit assessment protocols hinges on sustained, multiseason use of contextual metrics and psychological testing batteries to capture the influence of context on player performance and development over time. It is essential for sport organizations to track and understand their own influences on athletic performance over time. Organizational stress, perceptions of athlete, staff roles, and other features of performance environments have all been directly linked to athletic performance,[41–43] and, most importantly, following up on the success of performance fit indicators within and across seasons will serve to determine the predictive validity of the assessments used in drafts, enabling organizations to adapt and iteratively calibrate for high performance in a data-driven fashion.

Key Recommendations

Within the context of player selection, the authors recommend that a sports organization's management team, staff, psychologists/psychiatrists, and data scientists work together to achieve the following:

1. *Prioritize research and evaluation in the field of player selection.* The selection of high performing athletes is pivotal to many sports clubs and organizations. However, the empirical and theoretic underpinnings of athletic talent and performance in

applied settings have received little attention. Thus, there is a strong need for greater research and evaluation in the field of talent and "high performance" identification. Central to furthering such research and evaluation methodology, key stakeholders within the sport should create and defend their chosen standards and measurements, in accordance with their unique organization's culture, norms, and values of high performance.

2. *Caution the use of psychological assessment tools for categorizing individuals as "talented" versus "untalented."* Until validation methods for psychological testing batteries are improved across sporting contexts and can reliably predict future athletic performance, these measures should not be used to strictly categorize individuals as "talented" versus "untalented," or to "rule in" versus "rule out" players. Rather, the objective benefits that testing batteries provide should be harnessed within the broader ecological framework of the specific sports organization and position-specific demands to optimize assessment and development of high performance.

3. *Assess dynamic player-environment relations in selection assessment situations.* Organizations should make substantial efforts to evaluate "performance fit, the fit between a player's performance styles and the performance demands of the sporting environment. Ultimately, organizations that respect that high performance is as much a "state" that is continually and dynamically influenced by contexts as it is an acquired "trait" will be best positioned to identify and develop high performing athletes.

4. *Maintain a comprehensive database to track contextual factors and player performance metrics across seasons.* Organizations should clearly define and track metrics of performance contexts (eg, environmental conditions/resources, social and relational factors, position-specific demands) alongside their recruited players' game performance indicators in a sustained fashion. Over time, this can lead to the development of an organization-specific criterion model or athletic profile model that will enhance the ability to predict future athletic performance in an ecologically valid way.

COLLECTIVE DECISION MAKING

In the final process of collating all the information that has been gathered during the draft and forming final decisions regarding talent selection, it becomes imperative to know the process of selection: Who will be making the decision? What information do they need to know to inform that decision? What is the most effective way to present information to those who will be making the decision? It is best when talent selection can include multiple perspectives and multiple disciplines, especially if both objective and subjective data are being used. However, when multiple areas of expertise are used, it becomes increasingly important to create a clear process for gathering and communicating opinions. For instance, if a scout, a coach, or a team manager is tasked with athlete selection, the gathered information must be presented in a style and context that is understandable to them. Thus, a working understanding of the total information gathered and a shared language around communicating the findings and their significance are required. The psychologists and/or psychiatrists who are involved in the evaluation and selection process must provide education on both the benefits and the limitations of the different measures that were used, work with the selection team in developing a shared language, and collaborate with the other disciplines in creating a consistent framework. In addition, when selecting instruments for a psychological draft, a central goal of instrument selection should be to generate data that will help decision makers understand how bringing a certain player into the team may protect versus shift team dynamics and organizational culture. Ultimately, the authors do not advocate for professional sports organizations to use psychological assessment data as a screening tool that rules players in or out of selection based on specific player characteristics or attributes. Rather, they promote these techniques as a methodical assessment of "performance fit" between a player's performance characteristics, the team's organizational culture, and the inherent environmental demands of the position to be filled. Finally, a psychological draft evaluation should attempt to convey information to the decision makers about how resource intensive talent development may be: does the organization possess the necessary resources to invest to optimize performance fit for a prospective athlete? Subscribing to these core principles will increase the likelihood of an accurate contextualization of the psychological draft information that is provided and allow for the most informed talent selection decisions.

REFERENCES

1. Hunt AP, Orr RM, Billing DC. Developing physical capability standards that are predictive of success on special forces selection courses. Mil Med 2013; 178(6):619–24.
2. Lunt H. A pre-joining fitness test improves pass rates of Royal Navy recruits. Occup Med (Chic III) 2007;57:377–9.
3. Ranisavljev I, Mandic R, Cosic M, et al. NBA Pre-Draft Combine is the weak predictor of rookie basketball player's performance. J Hum Sport Exerc 2020; 16(3):1–10.
4. Woods CT, Joyce C, Robertson S. What are talent scouts actually identifying? Investigating the physical and technical skill match activity profiles of drafted and non-drafted U18 Australian footballers. J Sci Med Sport 2016;19(5):419–23.
5. Burgess D, Naughton G, Hopkins W. Draft-camp predictors of subsequent career success in the Australian Football League. J Sci Med Sport 2012;15(6):561–7.
6. Sierer PS, Battaglini CL, Mihalik JP, et al. The National Football League Combine: performance differences between drafted and nondrafted players entering the 2004 and 2005 drafts. J Strength Cond Res 2008;22(1):6–12.
7. Johnston K, Baker J. Waste reduction strategies: factors affecting talent wastage and the efficacy of talent selection in sport. Front Psychol 2020;10(January):1–11.
8. Woodward JR. Professional football scouts: an investigation of racial stacking. Sociology of Sport Journal 2004;21(4):356–75.
9. Lund S, Soderstrom T. To see or not to see: talent identification in the Swedish Football Association. Sociol Sport J 2017;34(3):248–58.
10. Bartone PT, Roland RR, Picano JJ, et al. Psychological hardiness predicts success in US Army Special Forces candidates. Int J Sel Assess 2008;16(1): 78–81. Available at: http://doi.wiley.com/10.1111/j.1468-2389.2008.00412.x. Accessed December 5, 2020.
11. De Beer M, Van Heerden A. Exploring the role of motivational and coping resources in a Special Forces selection process. SA Journal of Industrial Psychology 2014;40(1):1–3.
12. Smith EN, Young MD, Crum AJ, et al. Stress, mindsets, and success in Navy SEALs special warfare training. Front Psychol 2020;10(January):1–11.
13. Carless SA. Psychological testing for selection purposes: a guide to evidence-based practice for human resource professionals. The International Journal of Human Resource Management 2009;20(12):2517–32.

14. Bradbury T, Forsyth D. You're in; you're out: selection practices of coaches. An International Journal 2012.
15. Kinnunen T, Parviainen J. Feeling the right personality. Recruitment consultants' affective decision making in interviews with employee candidatesNordic journal of working life studies 2016;6(3):5–21.
16. Barrick MR, Shaffer JA, Degrassi SW. What you see may not be what you get: relationships among self-presentation tactics and ratings of interview and job performance. J Appl Psychol 2009;94(6):1394–411.
17. Guion RM. Assessment, measurement, and prediction for personnel decisions. 2nd edition. New York, NY: Taylor & Francis; 2011.
18. Finn SE, Tonsager ME. How therapeutic assessment became humanistic. Hum Psychol 2002;30(1–2):10–22.
19. Finn SE, Tbnsager ME. Information-gathering and therapeutic models of assessment: complementary paradigms. Psychol Assess 1997;9(4):374–85.
20. Kopp A, Jekauc D. The influence of emotional intelligence on performance in competitive sports: a meta-analytical investigation. Sports 2018;6(4):175.
21. Phillips E, Davids K, Renshaw I, et al. Expert performance in sport and the dynamics of talent development. Sports Med 2010;40(4):271–83.
22. Roffey K, Gross JB. A behavioural observation checklist for basketball talent identification. In: The 18th ACHPER National/International Conference Proceedings. 14-18 January 1991, Perth, Western Australia. p. 368–373.
23. Vaeyens R, Lenoir M, Williams AM, et al. Talent identification and development programmes in sport current models and future directions. Sports Med 2008; 38(9):703–14.
24. Elferink-gemser M, Visscher C, Lemmink K, et al. Relation between multidimensional performance characteristics and level of performance in talented youth field hockey players relation between multidimensional performance characteristics and level of performance in talented youth field hockey players. J Sports Sci 2011;22(11–12):1053–63.
25. Lyons BD, Hoffman BJ, Michel JW, et al. On the predictive efficiency of past performance and physical ability: the case of the National Football League on the predictive efficiency of past performance and physical ability: the case of the National Football League. Human Performance 2011;24(2):158–72.
26. Reilly T, Williams AM, Nevill A, et al. A multidisciplinary approach to talent identification in soccer. J Sports Sci 2000;18:695–702.
27. Anshel MH, Lidor R. Talent detection programs in sport: the questionable use of psychological measures. J Sport Behav 2012;35(3):239–66.
28. Abbott A, Button C, Zealand N, et al. Unnatural selection: talent identification and development in sport. Nonlinear Dyn Psychol Life Sci 2005;9(1):61–88.
29. Pinder RA, Renshaw I, Davids K. The role of representative design in talent development: a comment on "talent identification and promotion programmes of Olympic athletes. J Sports Sci 2013;31(8):803–6.
30. Den Hartigh RJR, Van Dijk MWG, Steenbeek HW. A dynamic network model to explain the development of excellent human performance. Front Psychol 2016; 7:1–20.
31. Ambrose D. Socioeconomic stratification and its influences on talent development: some interdisciplinary perspectives. Gifted Child Quarterly 2002;46(3):170–80.
32. Côté J, Abernethy B. A developmental approach to sport expertise. In: Murphy SM, editor. The Oxford handbook of sport and performance psychology. Oxford: Oxford University Press; 2012. p. 435–447.

33. Davids KW, Button C, Bennett SJ. Dynamics of skill acquisition: a constraints-led approach. Human Kinetics 2008.
34. Newell KM. Motor skill acquisition. Annual review of psychology 1991;42(1):213–37.
35. Newell KM, Mayer-kress G. Time scales in motor learning and development. Psychol Rev 2001;108(I):57–82.
36. Van Geert P. Dynamic systems of development: change between complexity and chaos. New York, NY: Harvester Wheatsheaf; 1994.
37. Bergkamp TLG, Niessen ASM, Den Hartigh RJR. Comment on: "talent identification in sport: a systematic review. Sport Med 2018;48(6):1517–9.
38. Bloom G. Role of the elite coach in the development of talent. In: Silva JM, Stevens EE, editors. Psychological foundations of sport. San Francisco: Benjamin-Cummings; 2002. p. 466–83.
39. Durand-bush N, Salmela JH. The development and maintenance of expert athletic performance: perceptions of world and Olympic champions of expert athletic performance. Journal of applied sport psychology 2002;14(3):154–71.
40. Iso-Ahola SE. Intrapersonal and interpersonal factors in athletic performance. Scand J Med Sci Sports 1995;5(4):191–9.
41. Fletcher D, Wagstaff CRD. Organizational psychology in elite sport: its emergence, application and future. Psychol Sport Exerc 2009;10(4):427–34.
42. Gould D, Maynard I. Psychological preparation for the Olympic games psychological preparation for the Olympic games. J Sports Sci 2009;27(13):1393–408.
43. Weinberg R, McDermott M. A comparative analysis of sport and business organizations: factors perceived critical for organizational success: a comparative analysis of sport and business organizations. J Appl Sport Psychol 2002;14:282–98.

Sport Psychiatry and Its Research Agenda

Alan Currie, MB ChB, MPhil, FRCPsych[a,b,c],*, Rosemary Purcell, BA, MPsych, PhD[d,e]

KEYWORDS

- Athletes • Sports • Sport Psychiatry • Mental health • Mental illness
- Mental disorders • Research

KEY POINTS

- More refined data are required on the prevalence and significance of mental health symptoms in sporting populations.
- The ecology of sport requires study for its potential contribution to the risk of developing mental health symptoms and disorders.
- The induction of athletes into elite sport is a neglected area of research.
- Evaluation is needed of the models of care best suited to elite sport.
- Evidence-based guidance is needed on "return to play" after a mental health problem.

INTRODUCTION

The agenda for Sport Psychiatry research arguably centers on one specific issue: are athletes "normal" individuals or are they different in some way, even unique? From this follows whether we can legitimately extrapolate the existing evidence base from general population studies or to what extent we must develop an athlete-specific understanding of the antecedents to mental health problems and their identification, treatment, and rehabilitation.

In seeking to understand the prevalence of mental health disorders in athlete populations, key questions emerge:

[a] Cumbria Northumberland Tyne and Wear NHS Foundation Trust, Regional Affective Disorders Service, Wolfson Research Centre, Campus for Ageing and Vitality, Westgate Road, Newcastle NE4 5PL, UK; [b] Mental Health Expert Panel (MHEP), English Institute of Sport, The Manchester Institute of Health and Performance, 299 Alan Turing Way, Manchester M11 3BS, UK; [c] Department of Sport and Exercise Science, University of Sunderland, City Campus, Sunderland SR1 3SD, UK; [d] Elite Sport and Mental Health, Orygen, 35 Poplar Road, Parkville, Victoria 3052, Australia; [e] Centre for Youth Mental Health, The University of Melbourne, Parkville Victoria 3052, Australia
* Corresponding author. Cumbria Northumberland Tyne and Wear NHS Foundation Trust, Regional Affective Disorders Service, Wolfson Research Centre, Campus for Ageing and Vitality, Westgate Road, Newcastle NE4 5PL, United Kingdom.
E-mail address: alan.currie@cntw.nhs.uk

Psychiatr Clin N Am 44 (2021) 493–505
https://doi.org/10.1016/j.psc.2021.04.007
0193-953X/21/Crown Copyright © 2021 Published by Elsevier Inc. All rights reserved.
psych.theclinics.com

- Are we entitled to rely on existing instruments developed for use in the general population or must we develop new and sports-specific tools?
- If we develop sports-specific measures, can we use the same instrument to survey every sport? For example, if a measure is valid in an aesthetic sport will it also be valid in an endurance event or a target sport?

Responding to mental health concerns in athletes currently relies heavily on extrapolating the evidence for treatments and therapies that has been developed and researched in the general population. Although we may not be able to replicate large randomized controlled trials in every sporting population, we need to know how to deliver psychotherapy to the itinerant athlete and we must understand how pharmacologic treatments interact with the athlete's physiology and performance.

Researching systems and models of care is also necessary and needs to address early identification and access to high-quality care. Services should also be evaluated on their ability to support the reintegration of athletes back into sport during recovery and in allowing an athlete to successfully leave sport, yet continue to enjoy the mental health benefits of physical activity and a life of participation.

This review is organized to consider gaps in research along a pathway that begins with prevalence studies and then considers prevention, screening, early detection, and early intervention, followed by treatment and rehabilitation before concluding with the athlete's departure from sport.

PREVALENCE

The prevalence of mental health symptoms among elite athletes has been examined in numerous cross-sectional surveys of self-reported symptoms. Gouttebarge and colleagues' systematic review and meta-analyses[1] provide the most comprehensive overview, indicating rates that range from 19% for alcohol misuse and 20% for psychological distress, through to 34% for anxiety/depression. Meta-analyses in former elite athletes indicate a broadly similar pattern of prevalence, with alcohol misuse (21%) and anxiety/depression (26%) particularly salient.

Most of the studies included in these meta-analyses involved nonrepresentative samples due to low survey response rates; this reduces confidence in the reported prevalence due to selection bias, where it is difficult to gauge whether or not athletes who are affected by mental ill health are more or less likely to respond to such surveys. Furthermore, the few included studies that involved "representative" samples consisted mostly of male athletes from professional team sports, which leaves the prevalence of symptoms in female athletes and athletes in individual sports and para-sports less well understood.

Studies published after Gouttebarge and colleagues' systematic review have addressed these limitations by examining more representative and/or inclusive elite athlete samples. A large survey of athletes from the Australian Institute of Sport (AIS) system (n = 749) involved participants who were representative of the eligible AIS population in terms of their age and para-status (although a somewhat higher proportion of female athletes participated). The rates of symptoms were as follows: 6% reported problematic gambling, 15% alcohol misuse, 18% "high to very high" psychological distress, 19.5% body and/or weight dissatisfaction, and 35% met the threshold for "probable caseness," which indicate a need for professional health care.[2] Compared with published community norms, the rates of psychological distress and "caseness" among athletes were higher, but the rates of problem gambling, risky alcohol consumption, and body dissatisfaction were significantly *lower*.[2] The prevalence of most mental health symptoms did not differ according to gender or para-status, with the exception of alcohol consumption, with the odds of misuse significantly lower in female athletes and para-athletes.

A study of 333 Swedish elite athletes (59% women) who had represented national teams in their sports in the past 3 years showed that 13% reported at least moderate levels of anxiety, 15% at least moderate levels of depressive symptoms, and 26% alcohol misuse.[3] The reported rates of anxiety and depression symptoms were significantly higher among female compared with male athletes, although the rates of alcohol misuse were similar.

Summary and Extension of the Research Agenda in Prevalence Studies

Mental health symptoms are sufficiently common in high-performance sport that sports medicine and allied health professionals are strongly encouraged to screen for mental health symptoms in elite athletes, in order to provide early detection and intervention. The IOC's Sports Mental Health Assessment Tool 1 (SMHAT-1)[4] has been recently developed for this specific purpose.

Gender differences in the reporting of mental health symptoms are increasingly evident and requires further research to elucidate their context and differential impacts on athletes. The rates of mental disorders in elite athletes are also underresearched and require future attention. Symptoms often fluctuate with sport-specific or other life stressors and may reflect high levels of subjective distress, but the extent to which this is accompanied by *functional impairment* is largely unknown. Understanding the rates of mental disorders in currently competing athletes and those transitioning out of sport is vital to establishing the need for more specialist care in elite sport settings and ensuring that athletes receive appropriate clinical interventions. Conducting high-quality research into the prevalence of mental disorders will be challenging, as reported rates will be biased in the absence of a representative sample, the latter being costly and difficult to assemble when standardized clinical interviews are necessary.

Research is also lacking in relation to the prevalence of mental ill health among coaches and support staff who are subject to many of the stressors encountered by elite athletes.[5] A recent study of coaches in New Zealand (n = 69; 77% male) found lower reported rates of depressive symptoms (14%) than those observed in both athletes and the general community,[6] although the odds of reporting symptoms were higher among coaches disclosing high levels of life stress and/or contemplating retirement. Because coaches play a vital role in helping to create "mentally healthy" environments for athletes and reducing stigma, research that better demonstrates their own mental health needs may help to "shift the needle" in relation to mental health obtaining parity with physical health in elite sport.

RISK FACTORS

Several sports-specific risk factors, as well as general life stressors are associated with mental ill health in elite athletes. The most robust risk factors across common mental health symptoms include severe or repetitive injury,[7,8] including concussion,[9] overtraining or insufficient recovery,[10] performance failure,[11] unplanned or involuntary retirement,[12] or in the case of athletes in para-sports, involuntary retirement due to declassification,[13] and transitions after major events, such as the Olympic Games.[14] Risk factors also vary across career phases, with harassment and abuse[15] and unsupportive or damaging relationships with parents and coaches particularly salient for the mental well-being of youth athletes.[16]

General risk factors include adverse life events,[1,2] inadequate social support or connectedness, and low self-esteem.[2,17] Age is also a consideration, given that the peak years of high-performance competition overlap with the primary ages of onset for many mental disorders.[18,19] There is scope for further research into a broader range of risk factors, including the impacts of social media and poor life balance, as well as an emphasis on *protective factors* for mental health and well-being.

Research into risk factors has focused predominantly at the level of the individual athlete or team; there is a paucity of research regarding *systemic factors* that influence mental health in sports. Research that takes account of the broader "ecology" of elite sporting environments is needed to advance understanding of these risk factors and the optimal responses required to address them.[20] This ecology extends beyond the athlete to encompass the "microsystem" of coaches and teammates and "macro-systems" such as individual sports and their national or international governing bodies (that may control funding or other levers that can affect athlete mental health). At the microsystem level for example, there is increasing research on the influence of coaching engagement and communication style on athlete psychological health and adaption to stress.[21] Examining risk factors within the broader ecological systems of elite sport is likely to be a fertile ground for future research.

PREVENTION

The transition *out* of sport has received far more attention than the transition *into* elite sport environments.[22,23] How sports can best "induct" athletes—as well as coaches and administrators—into sport in ways that ultimately promote mental health is a neglected area of research and potentially one of the more fruitful avenues to prevention.

Poor mental health literacy is well established as a barrier to help-seeking behavior in elite athletes,[24,25] which in turn reduces opportunities to prevent the onset of mental health symptoms or disorders. For example, eating disorder symptoms may go unnoticed in contexts where overexercising or restrictive eating habits are common.[26] Or an athlete may not be aware of the treatment options for eating disorders and incorrectly believe that disclosing their symptoms will result in hospitalization. Sports organizations are encouraged to offer mental health literacy programs to all athletes, coaches, and staff, tailored to developmental, cultural, social, and systemic issues related to sports.[27,28] The latter includes the consequences of seeking help such as potential loss of selection or income, which constitute major barriers and disincentives.[25] Mental health literacy training developed specifically for elite sport contexts shows promise,[29,30] although more research is needed as to whether such programs improve help-seeking *behavior* and not just intentions.[31]

SCREENING AND EARLY DETECTION

Universal screening of athletes for symptoms of, or risk factors for, common mental disorders may be an important approach to early identification,[32,33] but research suggests that this practice is seldom implemented.[34] Athlete-specific screening tools for detecting mental ill health may increase this practice and should be prioritized where possible,[35] such as the Athlete Psychological Strain Questionnaire[36] and the SMHAT-1,[4] although both of these measures require further validation and evaluation.

Any screening tools within elite sport settings must be used and interpreted by qualified and appropriately trained practitioners[33] with established procedures regarding when and to whom symptomatic or at-risk athletes will be referred.[37] Ethical practices are crucial for screening and early detection, as its purpose is *only* to identify the level of support required by athletes and/or to provide feedback to athletes to help promote improved self-awareness. Screening should not be used to exclude athletes based on mental ill health, particularly in the case of preparticipation or recruitment screening.

Critical times to screen include following severe injury (including concussion) and during the transition out of sports.[7] Further research is needed to determine the value of screening during the induction phase to high-performance sports (the "transition *in*" phase) and before and after major competitions, as well as which practitioners are best suited to conduct screening, including what credentials or training are needed to ensure safety and integrity in this process.[20]

EARLY INTERVENTION

Early interventions for mild to moderate mental ill health include low-cost and low-intensity approaches such as psychoeducation, problem-solving therapy, and mindfulness-based therapies.[20] Further study is required to determine the best modalities for delivering early interventions, including interventions at the individual, group, and/or team levels.

Beyond targeted psychological interventions, it is critical that early phase interventions also address issues related to the athlete's identity and the acquisition of interests and skills outside of sports, especially because these have a significant influence on mental health in the transitions out of sports.

Finally, early interventions are needed that encompass models of care that take into account the broad culture or ecology of sports, rather than the current and predominant approach where the individual athlete is the "identified patient."

TREATMENT
Psychological Interventions/Psychotherapy

There is good evidence for a wide range of psychotherapy interventions across a broad spectrum of mental health problems. These interventions include CBT and related treatments such as group CBT, computerized CBT, and CBT for eating disorders; interpersonal psychotherapy (IPT); acceptance and commitment therapy; brief dynamic psychotherapy; family therapy; behavioral couples therapy; and more. Athlete-specific research is negligible,[38] and athlete's psychotherapy is delivered based on extrapolating evidence from the general population.[39] It has been suggested that CBT is especially suited to athletes[40,41], and this observation warrants further investigation.

Delivery of psychotherapy by computer or via remote video link has received considerable attention as a response to the restrictions of a global pandemic.[42] These methods have particular appeal in elite sports and would overcome the difficulties of delivering therapy over a period of many weeks to an athlete who travels frequently (as many do) by a therapist who is not embedded within the team (as many are not). An important question is which therapies might be most deliverable by these means. For example, might therapies that can "manualize" (eg, CBT) be more effective when delivered at a distance than those that depend more on direct human interaction (eg, IPT or brief dynamic psychotherapy)? It has even been suggested that video consultations can offer advantages over conventional therapy sessions, for example, a therapy session for an athlete with an eating disorder during a meal or live exposure therapy for an athlete with an anxiety disorder.[42] This too warrants further study.

Among the stressors experienced by athletes are harassment, bullying, and even abuse.[15] Occasionally this is an individual issue but it is commonly experienced by multiple individuals within the same group and can go unacknowledged and unaddressed for long periods. Policies that prevent these abuses and that identify and arrest them at an early stage need to be augmented by an appropriate, validating, and supportive response for those affected.

Pharmacologic Treatments

The current approach to prescribing psychotropic medication for athletes is driven by expert consensus, delivered by the clinical judgment of the prescriber, and informed by the individual response (including tolerance of side effects) in the athlete.[43,44] It is described as "individualized prescribing" and includes addressing concerns about medication tolerability and its impact on performance. The large randomized controlled trials necessary to demonstrate a specific treatment effect in athlete populations are likely undeliverable with the small elite sporting samples available. However, the practice of extrapolating from general population evidence needs to be better informed by research in several areas.

Studies of the performance impact of antidepressant medication have involved small groups for short periods and often only include healthy subjects. Studies are required that replicate the use of these drugs in clinical practice and in particular their longer term use over weeks and months.[45] Adaptations in brain serotonin systems are complex, and changes seen within the first week after administration of selective serotonin reuptake inhibitor (SSRI) drugs are different from later changes that are thought to be responsible for the antidepressant response.[46] Studies should also include relevant measures of athletic performance alongside standard clinical symptom measures.[45] There is also a need to evaluate the effect of medication in groups that have been underrepresented in studies such as female athletes and athletes with disabilities. Antidepressants are not the only medication that could be prescribed for athletes, and other commonly used psychotropic medications too require study and in a similar way.[47] These medications include antipsychotic medication and mood stabilizers used in bipolar disorder, psychotic disorders, and occasionally in other situations such as treatment-resistant depression.

There are important steps that can be taken to increase the likelihood of benefit from, for example, antidepressant medication. Measurement-based care[48] and treatment delivered by algorithm[49] will both outperform "treatment as usual". Simple treatment pathways supported by algorithms lend themselves to the elite sports environment. For the itinerant athlete there is much that can be delivered remotely by the team doctor supported by a mental health expert such as a Sport Psychiatrist. These approaches warrant further evaluation specifically in sports.

The relationship between exercise and inflammation and between inflammation and depression requires further study in elite sporting populations. Immune function is suppressed temporarily by high-intensity exercise. In an overtrained athlete immune dysfunction may be more enduring,[50] and overtraining syndromes are frequently associated with depressive symptoms.[51,52] Increased inflammatory markers and altered immune function are also found in some depressive cohorts and may predict poor prognosis.[53] A different treatment approach may be needed when depression is associated with inflammation, as the usual first-line antidepressants drugs such as SSRIs may be less effective.[54] It has also been postulated that overtrained athletes benefit from rest, whereas depressed athletes experience an increase in symptoms in the same circumstances.[55] It would be useful to have this confirmed by further study.

RECOVERY, REHABILITATION, AND RETURN TO SPORTS

Many of the components of good mental health services for athletes have been described. Barriers to accessing services such as low levels of mental health literacy and the busy schedules of athletes need to be acknowledged and addressed.[24] Services are more likely to be used if they are on-site, free, and broad ranging.[56] The varied approaches of different countries and different sports to this have been reported.[33] Early intervention, cross-disciplinary collaboration, and targeted treatment of specific disorders have all been emphasized.[19] Future work requires that mental health services for athletes are evaluated and the results of these evaluations widely disseminated. Important questions include the following:

- What are the key elements of these services?
- How can a comprehensive service be adapted for low-income economies and settings?
- What constitutes a good outcome or outcomes for services in terms of both the health and performance of athletes?

Recovery, rehabilitation, and return to sports is a multidisciplinary endeavor and in particular requires close collaboration between sports medical staff, the clinical team delivering treatment, and the athlete's support team with the athlete involved in, and central to all decisions[57]; this is given particular emphasis in the case of injured athletes who may experience symptoms of poor mental health in close association with an injury and where rehabilitation and recovery are affected on both by the physical pathology of the injury and by mental health symptoms.[58]

Return-to-play criteria exist for many sports-related conditions.[59] Their development has been slower and more difficult in relation to mental health symptoms and disorders. Perhaps this reflects the relative paucity of objective and measurable data or pathology on which to base decisions and operationalize criteria. Return-to-play guidelines for eating disorders and related low energy availability[60–62] have been a welcome development and rely to a large extent on objective measures such as bone density, electrolyte disturbance, and electrocardiogram abnormalities. Expanding these guidelines to conditions such as depression, anxiety, and substance use disorders would be an important advance and could follow a similar template of red, amber, and green ratings according to the athlete's clinical condition.

After Sport

Leaving the sporting arena may mean relinquishing a strongly held sporting identity with little preparation to develop a new identity or identities.[63] Supporting athletes with this transition is important, and elements of this support have been described,[64] including the value of an "exit interview" focused on mental health.[1] Evaluating existing support programs is a priority. Identifying the most helpful elements will also allow focus where need is greatest, for example, those athletes who must make an abrupt transition after a career-ending injury or contract termination.

Some severe mental health problems may develop coincidently in elite sport; for example, the peak age of onset of bipolar and psychotic disorders overlaps closely with the ages of peak sporting performance.[33,47] For some who develop these conditions it may prove that they are incompatible with a continued career in elite sport. Because individuals with these disorders are at high risk of lifelong poor physical health and social exclusion,[47] it is important to support such athletes to continue in sports perhaps at a lower competitive level or in recreational/participative sport.

It has been suggested that retirement for athletes with disabilities is an especially difficult transition, as they move from being an inspiring role model to life away from sport and the stresses and disadvantages of a life with a disability.[65] Further study in this group of athletes is warranted, and a particular area to emphasize would be those whose retirement is enforced by reclassification that can mean retirement in circumstances that are perceived as subjective, arbitrary, and unfair.

Youth Sports

Mental health programs in sports often fail to target young athletes and are aimed only at elite performers.[66] Young and aspiring athletes may commit to training and competition and may have expectations placed on them that are very similar to the experiences of an elite athlete. There are also some sports where elite level participation is possible and not infrequent even at a very young age. The gaps in our knowledge of mental health in elite sport reflect the gaps evident in youth sport, but there are areas specific to youth sports that require particular investigation, which include how to match sporting practices and the sports culture most appropriately to the developmental stage of a young and developing athlete, especially if they are already competing in an adult world. Young athletes also need support to manage competing demands, most notably academic and sporting expectations.

Relevant frameworks for youth sports have been described[67] that emphasize the importance of an athlete-centered approach to ensure the various domains of the young athlete's personal functioning are developed, not only their sporting abilities. Treatment must also be tailored to the adolescent. This means that mental health and other professionals have appropriate training and registration to work with young athletes.[68] It also means that a broader range of psychotherapy interventions is available when needed, with more emphasis on systemic and especially family therapies.[69] Finally, adolescent athletes need support not only to transition into the elite sporting environment but also to leave sport and refocus their life if their ambitions are unfulfilled or their aspirations change.[47]

SUMMARY

This review began by asking to what extent existing knowledge and practice could be extrapolated into the environment of elite sport or to what extent sport-specific knowledge and practices were necessary. The answer inevitably is that both are relevant, important, and can be combined.

There is increasing knowledge of the prevalence of mental health symptoms in athletes; however, the significance of symptoms in the athletes requires greater understanding and more detailed investigation before we can accurately estimate the prevalence of disorders. Screening tools developed for use in the general population may be inadequate in sports or at least require interpretation that accounts for the ecology of sports, the demands on an athlete, and how these might influence the presentation of symptoms. Some subgroups require further study, most obviously female athletes, athletes with disabilities, younger athletes, and members of the athlete's entourage, including coaches.

Risk factors for the development of mental health symptoms that are specific to sports are increasingly understood. Mental health prevention work in sports needs to recognize this but must not be restricted by it and recognize that athletes are people and also subject to the same risk factors for the development of symptoms and disorders as the rest of the population. Improving mental health literacy requires that both perspectives are addressed: the athlete as a unique individual in unusual circumstances yet at the same time a normal human being.

Providing treatment of athletes would benefit from more emphasis on "how" rather than "what": how to deliver psychotherapy effectively in the unusual environment of elite sport and how to prescribe existing psychotropic medications safely and effectively with minimal performance impact. Primarily this necessitates not new therapies, new drugs, or sport-specific treatment trials but evaluation of existing treatments in an unusual context (elite sports).

The world of sports and the clinical world of health professionals should not be seen as separate or divided; this has general application across the field of sports and mental health, but most specifically in the need to collaborate to support an athlete during recovery, rehabilitation, and return to play. Return-to-play guidelines for a broader range of mental health symptoms and disorders are necessary. Templates for return-to-play guidance exist elsewhere in sports medicine, and their principles can be extrapolated for use in mental health conditions; this is not only practical but would ensure parity between mental and physical health.

The final element of comprehensive mental health services for athletes is in support for the exit from the elite sporting environment. As any retirement this is an adjustment with elements of loss and grief and requires reflection on developing a new identity, new activities, and sustaining a social support network. In sports, unlike other retirements, this process is often early, abrupt, unplanned, enforced, and complicated by factors such as injury. The value of both general and sport-specific understanding is once again emphasized.

There is much that is already known of mental health problems in elite sports, and our existing knowledge allows us to practice in a way that benefits the health and by extension the performance of the athlete. By acknowledging what we do not know, or need to refine, we can apply the sporting principles of continuous and incremental improvement in performance to shape the future of Sport Psychiatry practice.

CLINICS CARE POINTS

- Despite the mental health benefits of exercise, physical activity and sports participation, athletes will still experience mental health symptoms and disorders.
- Sports specific and general life stressors can contribute to the emergence of mental health symptoms and disorders in athletes.
- Aspects of the sports environments in which athletes train and compete can be both protective of, and contribute to the development and maintenance of mental health symptoms.
- Although treatment for athletes needs to account for their unique situation, the rationale for psychotherapy and pharmacologic interventions is still largely extrapolated from the evidence base that applies to the general population.

DECLARATIONS AND DISCLOSURE STATEMENT

The authors have nothing to disclose.

REFERENCES

1. Gouttebarge V, Castaldelli-Maia JM, Gorczynski P, et al. Occurrence of mental health symptoms and disorders in current and former elite athletes: A systematic review and meta-analysis. Br J Sports Med 2019;53(11):700–6.
2. Purcell R, Rice S, Butterworth M, et al. Rates and Correlates of Mental Health Symptoms in Currently Competing Elite Athletes from the Australian National High-Performance Sports System. Sports Med 2020. https://doi.org/10.1007/s40279-020-01266-z.

3. Åkesdotter C, Kenttä G, Eloranta S, et al. The prevalence of mental health problems in elite athletes. J Sci Med Sport 2020;23(4):329–35.

4. Gouttebarge V, Bindra A, Blauwet C, et al. International Olympic Committee (IOC) Sport Mental Health Assessment Tool 1 (SMHAT-1) and Sport Mental Health Recognition Tool 1 (SMHRT-1): towards better support of athletes' mental health. Br J Sports Med 2020;0:1–9.

5. Olusoga P, Butt J, Hays K, et al. Stress in elite sports coaching: Identifying stressors. J Appl Sport Psychol 2009;21(4):442–59.

6. Kim SSY, Hamiliton B, Beable S, et al. Elite coaches have a similar prevalence of depressive symptoms to the general population and lower rates than elite athletes. BMJ Open Sport Exerc Med 2020;6(1). https://doi.org/10.1136/bmjsem-2019-000719.

7. Reardon CL, Hainline B, Aron CM, et al. Mental health in elite athletes: International Olympic Committee consensus statement (2019). Br J Sports Med 2019;53(11):667–99.

8. Chang C, Putukian M, Aerni G, et al. Mental health issues and psychological factors in athletes: Detection, management, effect on performance and prevention: American Medical Society for Sports Medicine Position Statement-Executive Summary. Br J Sports Med 2020;54(4):216–20.

9. Rice SM, Gwyther K, Santesteban-Echarri O, et al. Determinants of anxiety in elite athletes: a systematic review and meta-analysis. Br J Sports Med 2019;53(11):722–30.

10. Frank R, Nixdorf I, Beckmann J. Depression in elite athletes: Prevalence and psychological factors. Dtsch Z Sportmed 2013;64(11):320–6.

11. Hammond T, Gialloreto C, Kubas H, et al. The prevalence of failure-based depression among elite athletes. Clin J Sports Med 2013;23(4):273–7.

12. Park S, Lavallee D, Tod D. Athletes' career transition out of sport: A systematic review. Int Rev Sport Exerc Psychol 2013;6(1):22–53.

13. Bundon A, Ashfield A, Smith B, et al. Struggling to stay and struggling to leave: The experiences of elite para-athletes at the end of their sport careers. Psychol Sport Exerc 2018;37:296–305.

14. Howells K, Lucassen M. 'Post-Olympic blues' –The diminution of celebrity in Olympic athletes. Psychol Sport Exerc 2018;37:67–78.

15. Mountjoy M, Brackenridge C, Arrington M, et al. International Olympic Committee consensus statement: Harassment and abuse (non-accidental violence) in sport. Br J Sports Med 2016;50(17):1019–29.

16. Sabato T, Walch T, Caine D. The elite young athlete: strategies to ensure physical and emotional health. Open Access J Sports Med 2016;7:99–113.

17. Armstrong S, Oomen-Early J. Social connectedness, self-esteem, and depression symptomatology among collegiate athletes versus nonathletes. J Am Coll Heal 2009;57(5):521–6.

18. Kessler RC, Berglund P, Demler O, et al. Lifetime prevalence and age-of-onset distributions of DSM-IV disorders in the national comorbidity survey replication. Arch Gen Psychiatry 2005;62(6):593–602.

19. Rice SM, Purcell R, De Silva S, et al. The Mental Health of Elite Athletes: A Narrative Systematic Review. Sports Med 2016;46(9):1333–53.

20. Purcell R, Gwyther K, Rice SM. Mental Health In Elite Athletes: Increased Awareness Requires An Early Intervention Framework to Respond to Athlete Needs. Sports Med Open 2019;5(1):46–54.

21. Burns L, Weissensteiner JR, Cohen M. Supportive interpersonal relationships: A key component to high-performance sport. Br J Sports Med 2019;53(22): 1387–90.
22. Bruner MW, Munroe-Chandler KJ, Spink KS. Entry into elite sport: A preliminary investigation into the transition experiences of rookie athletes. J Appl Sport Psychol 2008;20(2):236–52.
23. Stambulova NB, Ryba TV, Henriksen K. Career development and transitions of athletes: the International Society of Sport Psychology Position Stand Revisited. Int J Sport Exerc Psychol 2020;1–27. https://doi.org/10.1080/1612197X.2020. 1737836.
24. Castaldelli-Maia JM, Gallinaro JGDME, Falcão RS, et al. Mental health symptoms and disorders in elite athletes: A systematic review on cultural influencers and barriers to athletes seeking treatment. Br J Sports Med 2019;53(11):707–21.
25. Gulliver A, Griffiths KM, Christensen H. Barriers and facilitators to mental health help-seeking for young elite athletes: a qualitative study. BMC Psychiatry 2012; 12(1):157.
26. Joy E, Kussman A, Nattiv A. 2016 update on eating disorders in athletes: A comprehensive narrative review with a focus on clinical assessment and management. Br J Sports Med 2016;50(3):154–62.
27. Gorczynski P, Currie A, Gibson K, et al. Developing mental health literacy and cultural competence in elite sport. J Appl Sport Psychol 2020. https://doi.org/10. 1080/10413200.2020.1720045.
28. Van Slingerland KJ, Durand-Bush N, Bradley L, et al. Canadian Centre for Mental Health and Sport (CCMHS) Position Statement: Principles of Mental Health in Competitive and High-Performance Sport. Clin J Sports Med 2019;29(3):173–80.
29. Purcell R, Chevroulet C, Pilkington V, et al. What works for mental health in sporting teams? An evidence guide for best practice in mental health promotion and early intervention. Orygen, Melbourne; 2020.
30. Sebbens J, Hassmén P, Crisp D, et al. Mental Health in Sport (MHS): Improving the Early Intervention Knowledge and Confidence of Elite Sport Staff. Front Psychol 2016;7(JUN):911.
31. Liddle SK, Deane FP, Batterham M, et al. A brief sports-based mental health literacy program for male adolescents: a cluster-randomized controlled trial. J Appl Sport Psychol 2019. https://doi.org/10.1080/10413200.2019.1653404.
32. Kroshus E. Variability in institutional screening practices related to collegiate student-athlete mental health. J Athl Train 2016;51(5):389–97.
33. Moesch K, Kenttä G, Kleinert J, et al. FEPSAC position statement: Mental health disorders in elite athletes and models of service provision. Psychol Sport Exerc 2018;38(January):61–71.
34. Sudano LE, Miles CM. Mental Health Services in NCAA Division I Athletics: A Survey of Head ATCs. Sports Health 2017;9(3):262–7.
35. Henriksen K, Schinke R, Moesch K, et al. Consensus statement on improving the mental health of high performance athletes. Int J Sport Exerc Psychol 2019. https://doi.org/10.1080/1612197x.2019.1570473.
36. Rice SM, Parker AG, Mawren D, et al. Preliminary psychometric validation of a brief screening tool for athlete mental health among male elite athletes: the Athlete Psychological Strain Questionnaire. Int J Sport Exerc Psychol 2019;1–16. https://doi.org/10.1080/1612197X.2019.1611900.
37. Gearity B, Moore EWG, Sharp C. National Strength and Conditioning Association's Endorsement of the National Collegiate Athletic Association Sport Science Institute's "mental Health Best Practices: Inter-Association Consensus Document:

Best Practices for Understanding and Supporting Stu. Strength Cond J 2017; 39(4):1–3.

38. Stillman MA, Glick ID, McDuff D, et al. Psychotherapy for mental health symptoms and disorders in elite athletes: A narrative review. Br J Sports Med 2019;53(12): 767–71.

39. Glick ID, Stillman MA, Reardon CL, et al. Managing Psychiatric Issues in Elite Athletes. J Clin Psychiatry 2012;73(05):640–4.

40. Hays K. Working it out: using exercise in psychotherapy. In: Hays K, editor. Washington, DC: American Psychological Association Inc.; 1999. p. 177–87.

41. Stillman MA, Ritvo EC, Glick ID. Psychotherapeutic Treatment of Athletes and their Significant Others. In: Baron DA, Reardon CL, Baron SH, editors. Clinical sports psychiatry: an international perspective. Oxford: Wiley-Blackwell; 2013. p. 117–23.

42. Reardon CL, Bindra A, Blauwet C, et al. Mental health management of elite athletes during COVID-19: a narrative review and recommendations. Br J Sports Med 2020;1–10. https://doi.org/10.1136/bjsports-2020-102884.

43. Johnston A, McAllister-Williams RH. Psychotropic Drug Prescribing. In: Currie A, Owen B, editors. Sports psychiatry. 1st edition. Oxford: Oxford University Press; 2016. p. 133–43.

44. Reardon CL, Creado S. Psychiatric medication preferences of sports psychiatrists. Physician Sports Med 2016;44(4):397–402.

45. Reardon CL, Factor R. The use of psychiatric medication by athletes. In: Baron DA, Reardon CL, Baron SH, editors. Clinical sports psychiatry: an international perspective. Oxford: Wiley-Blackwell; 2013. p. 157–62.

46. Fritze S, Spanagel R, Noori HR. Adaptive dynamics of the 5-HT systems following chronic administration of selective serotonin reuptake inhibitors: a meta-analysis. J Neurochem 2017;142(5):747–55.

47. Currie A, Gorczynski P, Rice SM, et al. Bipolar and psychotic disorders in elite athletes: a narrative review. Br J Sports Med 2019;53(12):746–53.

48. Guo T, Xiang YT, Xiao L, et al. Measurement-based care versus standard care for major depression: A randomized controlled trial with blind raters. Am J Psychiatry 2015;172(10):1004–13.

49. Bauer M, Pfennig A, Linden M, et al. Efficacy of an algorithm-guided treatment compared with treatment as usual: A randomized, controlled study of inpatients with depression. J Clin Psychopharmacol 2009;29(4):327–33.

50. Gleeson M. Immune function in sport and exercise. J Appl Physiol 2007;103(2): 693–9.

51. Armstrong LE, VanHeest JL. The unknown mechanism of the overtraining syndrome: clues from depression and psychoneuroimmunology. Sports Med 2002; 32(3):185–209. Available at: http://www.ncbi.nlm.nih.gov/pubmed/11839081. Accessed October 15, 2016.

52. Schwenk TL. The stigmatisation and denial of mental illness in athletes. Br J Sports Med 2000;34(1):4–5.

53. Miller AH. Beyond depression: the expanding role of inflammation in psychiatric disorders. World Psychiatry 2020;19(1):108–9.

54. Uher R, Maier W, Hauser J, et al. Differential efficacy of escitalopram and nortriptyline on dimensional measures of depression. Br J Psychiatry 2009;194(3): 252–9.

55. Reardon CL, Factor RM. Sport Psychiatry: A systematic review of diagnosis and medical treatment of mental illness in athletes. Sports Med 2010;40(11):961–80.

56. McDuff DR, Garvin M. Working with sports organizations and teams. Int Rev Psychiatry 2016;28(6):595–605.
57. Currie A, Johnston A. Psychiatric disorders: The psychiatrist's contribution to sport. Int Rev Psychiatry 2016;28(6):587–94.
58. Putukian M. The psychological response to injury in student athletes: a narrative review with a focus on mental health. Br J Sports Med 2016;50(3):145–8.
59. Herring SA, Kibler W Ben, Putukian M. The team physician and the return-to-play decision: a consensus statement-2012 update. Med Sci Sports Exerc 2012;44(12):2446–8.
60. Joy E, De Souza MJ, Nattiv A, et al. 2014 Female athlete triad coalition consensus statement on treatment and return to play of the female athlete triad. Curr Sports Med Rep 2014;13(4):219–32.
61. Mountjoy M, Sundgot-Borgen J, Burke L, et al. The IOC consensus statement: beyond the Female Athlete Triad-Relative Energy Deficiency in Sport (RED-S). Br J Sports Med 2014;48(7):491–7.
62. Mountjoy M, Sundgot-Borgen JK, Burke LM, et al. IOC consensus statement on relative energy deficiency in sport (RED-S): 2018 update. Br J Sports Med 2018;52(11):687–97.
63. Lavallee D, Robinson HK. In pursuit of an identity: A qualitative exploration of retirement from women's artistic gymnastics. Psychol Sport Exerc 2007;8(1):119–41.
64. Knights S, Sherry E, Ruddock-Hudson M. Investigating Elite End-of-Athletic-Career Transition: A Systematic Review. J Appl Sport Psychol 2016;28(3):291–308.
65. Swartz L, Hunt X, Bantjes J, et al. Mental health symptoms and disorders in Paralympic athletes: A narrative review. Br J Sports Med 2019;53(12):737–40.
66. Hill A, Macnamara Á, Collins D, et al. Examining the Role of Mental Health and Clinical Issues within Talent Development. Front Psycholgy 2016;6:1–11.
67. Vella SA. Mental Health and Organized Youth Sport. Kinesiol Rev 2019;8(3):229–36.
68. Breslin G, Smith A, Donohue B, et al. International consensus statement on the psychosocial and policy-related approaches to mental health awareness programmes in sport. BMJ Open Sport Exerc Med 2019;1–7. https://doi.org/10.1136/bmjsem-2019-000585.
69. National Institute for Health and Care Excellence. Eating disorders: recognition and treatment. NICE Guidel. 2017;(May):1-40. Available at: https://www.nice.org.uk/guidance/ng69/resources/eating-disorders-recognition-and-treatment-pdf-1837582159813. Accessed December 16, 2020.

Moving?

Make sure your subscription moves with you!

To notify us of your new address, find your **Clinics Account Number** (located on your mailing label above your name), and contact customer service at:

Email: journalscustomerservice-usa@elsevier.com

800-654-2452 (subscribers in the U.S. & Canada)
314-447-8871 (subscribers outside of the U.S. & Canada)

Fax number: 314-447-8029

Elsevier Health Sciences Division
Subscription Customer Service
3251 Riverport Lane
Maryland Heights, MO 63043

*To ensure uninterrupted delivery of your subscription, please notify us at least 4 weeks in advance of move.

Printed and bound by CPI Group (UK) Ltd, Croydon, CR0 4YY

03/10/2024

01040400-0016